W9-BUD-344

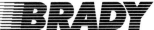

WORKBOOK
Scott Vahradian

FIRST RESPONDER

A Skills Approach

FIFTH EDITION

Keith J. Karren, Ph.D.
Chair, Department of Health Sciences
Brigham Young University
Provo, Utah

Brent Q. Hafen, Ph.D.
Professor, Department of Health Sciences
Brigham Young University
Provo, Utah

Daniel Limmer, EMT-P
Paramedic, Colonie EMS Department, Colonie, New York
Training Officer, Colonie Police Department, Colonie, New York
Instructor, Hudson Valley Community College, Institute of Prehospital Emergency Medicine, Troy, New York

Medical Editor
Edward T. Dickinson, M.D., FACEP

BRADY
PRENTICE HALL, UPPER SADDLE RIVER, NEW JERSEY 07458

Contributor:
Deborah A. Kufs, B.S., R.N., NREMT-P
Clinical Instructor, Hudson Valley Community
College, Institute of Prehospital Emergency Medicine,
Troy, New York

Publisher: Susan Katz
Marketing Manager: Judy Streger
Managing Production Editor: Patrick Walsh
Production Liaison: Julie Boddorf
Managing Development Editor: Lois Berlowitz
Development Editor: Josephine Cepeda
Associate Editor: Arlene Bregman
Production Editor/Interior Design: Barbara J. Barg,
    Navta Associates, Inc.
Cover Design: Bruce Kenselaar
Cover Photography:
    Photo Left: Howard M. Paul, Emergency! Stock
    Photo Center: Michael Gallitelli
    Photo Right: Michal Heron
Director of Manufacturing & Production:
    Bruce Johnson
Manufacturing Buyer: Ilene Sanford
Editorial Assistant: Carol Sobel

©1998 by Prentice-Hall, Inc.
A Simon & Schuster Company
Upper Saddle River, New Jersey 07458

*All rights reserved. No part of this book may be repro-
duced, in any form or by any means, without permission
in writing from the publisher.*

Printed in the United States of America

10 9 8 7 6 5 4 3 2 1

ISBN 0-8359-5143-X

Prentice Hall International (UK) Limited, *London*
Prentice Hall of Australia Pty., Limited, *Sydney*
Prentice Hall Canada Inc., *Toronto*
Prentice Hall Hispanoamericana, S.A., *Mexico*
Prentice Hall of India Private Limited, *New Delhi*
Prentice Hall of Japan, *Tokyo*
Simon & Schuster Asia Pte. Ltd., *Singapore*
Editora Prentice Hall do Brasil, Ltda., *Rio de Janeiro*

NOTICE ON CARE PROCEDURES

It is the intent of the authors and publisher that this workbook be used as part of a formal First Responder education program taught by qualified instructors and supervised by a licensed physician. The procedures described in this workbook are based upon consultation with First Responder and medical authorities. The authors and publisher have taken care to make certain that these procedures reflect currently accepted clinical practice; however, they cannot be considered absolute recommendations.

The material in this workbook contains the most current information available at the time of publication. However, federal, state, and local guidelines concerning clinical practices, including, without limitation, those governing infection control and universal precautions, change rapidly. The reader should note, therefore, that new regulations may require changes in some procedures.

It is the responsibility of the reader to familiarize himself or herself with the policies and procedures set by federal, state, and local agencies as well as the institution or agency where the reader is employed. The authors and the publisher of this workbook disclaim any liability, loss, or risk resulting directly or indirectly from the suggested procedures and theory, from any undetected errors, or from the reader's misunderstanding of the text. It is the reader's responsibility to stay informed of any new changes or recommendations made by any federal, state, and local agency as well as by his or her employing institution or agency.

CONTENTS

MODULE 1: PREPARATORY

MODULE 2: AIRWAY

MODULE 3: CIRCULATION

MODULE 4: PATIENT ASSESSMENT

MODULE 5: ILLNESS AND INJURY

MEDICAL EMERGENCIES

BLEEDING AND SOFT-TISSUE INJURIES

INJURIES TO MUSCLES AND BONES

MODULE 6: CHILDBIRTH AND CHILDREN

MODULE 7: EMS OPERATIONS

CHAPTER 1

INTRODUCTION TO THE EMS SYSTEM

KEY IDEAS

This chapter provides an overview of the EMS system and the roles and responsibilities of the First Responder in the EMS system. Key ideas include the following:

- The EMS system is a network of resources linked together for the purpose of providing emergency care and transport to victims of sudden illness and injury.

- The public has access to the EMS system through 9-1-1 and non-9-1-1 phone numbers.

- There are four levels of EMS training: First Responder, EMT-Basic, EMT-Intermediate, and EMT-Paramedic.

- The First Responder is the first person with emergency medical training on the scene of a sudden injury or illness.

- First Responders are the designated agents of the medical director, who is the physician responsible for out-of-hospital emergency medical care.

CONTENT REVIEW

1. The emergency medical services (EMS) system is organized to:
   a. provide care to victims of sudden illness or injury.
   b. deny non-emergency personnel access to the scene.
   c. coordinate extrication and rescue operations.
   d. upgrade 9-1-1 phone systems all over the U.S.

2. The National Highway Traffic Safety Administration recommends that every EMS system include 10 basic components. Write a brief description of each component:

   a. Regulation and policy:

   b. Resources management:

   c. Human resources and training:

   d. Transportation:

   e. Facilities:

   f. Communications:

   g. Public information and education:

   h. Medical oversight:

   i. Trauma systems:

   j. Evaluation:

3. There are two general systems by which the public can access EMS. They are 9-1-1 and non-9-1-1 systems.

_____ True

_____ False

4. List the four levels of out-of-hospital care providers.

a.

b.

c.

d.

5. First Responders are the first:
   a. law enforcement officials on scene.
   b. people with emergency medical training.
   c. rescuers who can administer medications.
   d. people to notice that an emergency exists.

6. A _____ is a medical facility that specializes in the care of injuries to a patient's body.
   a. trauma center
   b. pediatric center
   c. poison control center
   d. local hospital emergency department

7. What is your role as a First Responder? List eight tasks you should perform.

a.

b.

c.

d.

e.

f.

g.

h.

8. One of your responsibilities as a First Responder is to guard your own health and safety. Identify the item(s) below that are consistent with that responsibility.
   a. Drive safely at all times.
   b. Do not enter high traffic areas.
   c. Use a seat belt whenever you drive or ride.
   d. Enter a crime scene after you see the criminal leave it.
   e. Remove yourself from gas leaks and other such hazards.
   f. Always wear the appropriate personal protective equipment.

9. The EMS medical director is responsible for providing guidance to all emergency care and rescue personnel.

   _____ True

   _____ False

10. An EMS medical director is a physician who oversees EMS care of patients in the field in two ways:
    a. directly and indirectly.
    b. horizontally and vertically.
    c. out-of-hospital assessment and treatment.
    d. prescription and administration of medication.

11. Write an example for each type of medical control listed below.

    a. Direct medical control:

    b. Indirect medical control:

12. A First Responder is considered to be an extension of the _____

    _____ authority.

13. Maintaining a clean, professional appearance is nice but not a realistic goal for a First Responder.

    _____ True

    _____ False

14. It is the First Responder's responsibility to meet the standard of care with all patients, no matter their gender, age, culture, or socioeconomic background.

    _____ True

    _____ False

CASE STUDY:
FIRST ON SCENE

Read this scenario and answer the questions that follow. Focus on your role/responsibilities as a First Responder.

You and your partner have just completed the evening check of your equipment, when the dispatcher sends your unit to a man having "difficulty breathing" at a restaurant. When you arrive in front of the small restaurant, there is a group of very worried patrons at the curb. They tell you that the patient, Mr. Gianelli, must be having a heart attack. They say he cannot breathe well and is clutching his chest and neck. When you determine that it is safe to do so, you leave your vehicle, enter the restaurant, and approach Mr. Gianelli.

15. Should you act on the bystander information that Mr. Gianelli is having a heart attack? Explain your answer.

At Mr. Gianelli's side, you assess that he is awake, that he cannot speak or breathe, and that this happened while eating steak and laughing. Your partner performs a Heimlich maneuver on Mr Gianelli, immediately expelling the bit of food that was blocking his airway. Mr. Gianelli can now breathe. His voice is very hoarse.

16. What are your roles/responsibilities now? Name at least three.

17. The EMTs arrive to continue patient care and transport. What are your roles and responsibilities now? Name at least three.

CHAPTER 2

THE WELL-BEING OF THE FIRST RESPONDER

KEY IDEAS

This chapter outlines the basic steps you should take to maintain your well-being. It discusses how to anticipate and handle the emotional aspects of emergencies. It also introduces you to scene safety, including how to protect yourself against infection. Key ideas are as follows:

- Death and dying are inherent parts of emergency medical care. When your patient is dying, you must care for his or her emotional needs as well as the injury or illness. If the patient dies suddenly, help the family or bystanders deal with their grief.

- The five stages of the grieving process are denial, anger, bargaining, depression, and acceptance.

- Stress related to EMS work can have a negative affect on First Responders. Be aware of the warning signs. Lifestyle changes—including keeping physically fit and maintaining a balance between work and family—can help you deal with stress effectively.

- Critical incident stress requires aggressive and immediate management. One way to meet that need is through a critical incident stress debriefing, a process by which a team of peer counselors and mental health professionals help rescuers deal with their feelings.

- Another way First Responders protect themselves in the field is by preventing infection by disease. In order to do that successfully, you must practice a strict form of infection control—body substance isolation (BSI)—with all patients. You also must clean, disinfect, or sterilize your equipment properly. Also follow your physician's orders in regard to immunizations.

- It is imperative that you do not fall victim to the same problems that affect your patients. Therefore, do not enter the scene of an emergency until you have determined it is safe to do so. If the scene is unsafe, make it safe before you enter.

CONTENT REVIEW

▼

1. Identify the items below that describe high-stress situations.
   a. A patient in your care stops breathing.
   b. A hit-and-run involves an eight-year-old boy.
   c. You hear that a coworker has died on the job.
   d. You suspect physical abuse of a patient in your care.
   e. A two-car collision results in injury to four adults.
   f. A factory worker just had part of his hand amputated.
   g. You hear loud, angry voices in the apartment to which you were called.

2. What are some immediate strategies you can use to lessen the effects of an emotional response to a high-stress situation?

   a.

   b.

   c.

   d.

3. Dying patients—and those close to them—experience what is called the "grieving process." This process includes five stages, which are:
   a. anger, acceptance, sorrow, shock, despair.
   b. shock, silence, acceptance, anger, mourning.
   c. denial, rage, blame, forgiveness, acceptance.
   d. denial, anger, bargaining, depression, acceptance.

4. One way a First Responder can help a dying patient's family is by:
   a. keeping them away from the dying patient.
   b. allowing them to cry and get angry, even at you.
   c. gently assuring them that everything will be all right.
   d. saying as little as possible about the patient's condition.

5. Dealing with chronic stress may require a First Responder to make some lifestyle changes. List four examples.

   a.

   b.

   c.

   d.

6. As a First Responder, the members of your family may suffer from stress related to your job, too. Describe four of their possible stress factors.

   a.

   b.

   c.

   d.

7. Any event that causes unusually strong emotions, which interfere with your ability to function either during an emergency or later, is called a:
   a. burnout.
   b. mental breakdown.
   c. critical incident.
   d. crisis of conscience.

8. A critical incident stress debriefing may include:
   a. only EMS workers who were at the scene.
   b. anyone involved in the critical incident.
   c. disaster support services personnel only.
   d. the rescue workers, not the commanders.

9. One CISD technique is called "defusing." It is _____ than a debriefing.
   a. shorter and less formal
   b. longer and more formal
   c. shorter and more formal
   d. longer and less formal

10. A critical incident stress debriefing is usually held _____ the incident.
    a. 30 to 45 minutes after
    b. 30 to 45 minutes before
    c. 24 to 72 hours before
    d. 24 to 72 hours after

11. List six circumstances for which a First Responder would access CISD.

    a.

    b.

    c.

    d.

    e.

    f.

12. An infectious disease can spread *directly* from person to person by way of all of the following EXCEPT:
    a. blood-to-blood contact.
    b. contact with mucous membranes.
    c. a contaminated object such as a needle.
    d. contact with open wounds or exposed tissues.

13. Which of the following is NOT true of hepatitis B?
    a. It directly affects the liver.
    b. It can last for months, and it can be fatal.
    c. It is contracted through intimate contact only.
    d. An infected person may not know he or she has it.

14. When you are caring for a patient who might have tuberculosis, protect yourself against infection by:
    a. wearing an OSHA-approved respirator.
    b. avoiding any kind of artificial ventilation.
    c. turning your face away when the patient coughs.
    d. having contact only with the patient's clothing.

15. Transmission of HIV, the AIDS virus, requires intimate contact with the body fluids of an infected person. That means infection may occur in all of the following circumstances EXCEPT which two?
    a. changing an infected baby's diaper
    b. using infected blood in a transfusion
    c. during pregnancy, from mother to child
    d. injecting an infected needle into your skin
    e. sharing a warm drink with an infected person
    f. sexual contact involving the exchange of semen

16. The single most important thing you can do to prevent the spread of infection is to:
    a. get vaccinations and booster shots.
    b. wash your hands after caring for a patient.
    c. wear gloves with all patients no matter what.
    d. clean, disinfect, or sterilize your equipment.

17. The term "body substance isolation" refers to a strict form of infection control in which you assume that:
    a. where there's smoke there's fire.
    b. only blood can transmit fatal diseases.
    c. all patients who seem to be ill are ill.
    d. all blood and body fluids are infectious.

18. Describe the personal protective equipment appropriate for each of the following emergencies.

a. An unresponsive elderly man who is lying on a bed wet with urine.

b. A 16-year-old girl has been stabbed in her thigh. The blood is spurting out with force.

c. A 24-year-old male who is complaining of a painful, swollen ankle after tripping over a curb. No blood or other body fluids are present.

d. A 72-year-old woman on her living room floor who is not breathing and has no pulse.

e. A six-year-old with a shallow two-inch cut in his lower leg. A moderate amount of bleeding is present. The blood is oozing, rather than spurting.

19. For patients with diseases for which you have been vaccinated, you do not have to take BSI precautions.

_____ True

_____ False

20. Listed below are descriptions of five emergency scenes. Decide whether or not you would enter each one. Write "yes" or "no" in the space provided.

_____ **a.** You happen across an auto wreck and find two moderately injured patients trapped in a sedan. Right beside the car is a downed power line. It does not appear to be "hot."

_____ **b.** You are out one Saturday night catching a show at a nightclub when a fight breaks out just outside the front entrance. A woman screams that somebody has been stabbed. You step outside to find a large group of people gathered a short distance away. There is much screaming and shouting. The patient appears to be at the center of this group.

_____ **c.** You are waiting on a customer in your hardware store when a passerby runs in and shouts that the office building next to yours is on fire. You run out to investigate and find that smoke is billowing out of open windows and doors.

_____ **d.** You arrive at the scene of an assault. The assailant has reportedly fled, and law enforcement officers state that they have secured the scene. They want you to look at the assault victim.

_____ **e.** A chemical tanker has overturned on the interstate. You arrive and are told that a small amount of the chemical has spilled. The local fire department has begun to contain the spill. There is one critically injured patient who is lying on the ground about 10 feet from the spill.

CASE STUDY:
THE AIDS PATIENT
▼

Read this scenario and answer the questions that follow. Focus on strategies you can use to protect yourself and your coworkers from infectious exposure.

It's late on a Tuesday night, and you are responding in your private vehicle to a "man down" at a residence. You arrive at the scene and note that two other responders' units are parked on the street. You enter the home and find them assessing the patient in a back bedroom. The patient is 42 years old. He states that he was diagnosed with AIDS 15 months ago and was recently prescribed some medication that has been making him nauseous. This evening he threw up four times, and then may have passed out. He states that his vomit looked "a little bloody." He is pale and sweaty. Small amounts of vomit cling to his bathrobe. He also states that he is moderately short of breath, a problem associated with a recent "flu."

21. What specific sources of infectious exposure are you concerned about with this patient?

22. What personal protective gear will you wear when managing this patient?

As you begin to assist the other First Responders, you notice that one of them is not wearing protective gear. You have the opportunity to question her about this a short while later, and she states, "Look. I know that this guy has AIDS, but it's not like there's blood everywhere. I'm watching where I put my hands, so relax."

23. Critique her argument. Do you agree with her rationale? Disagree? Explain your answer.

24. You assist paramedics in transporting this patient to the hospital. En route, he vomits twice more and you see it contains a small amount of blood. After turning the patient over to the emergency department team, what steps would you then take to eliminate possible contamination?

CHAPTER 3

LEGAL AND ETHICAL ISSUES

KEY IDEAS

This chapter describes your scope of practice and what it means to have a duty to act. It defines patient consent and explains advance directives. It also gives you an overview of various other legal issues that will affect you in the field. Key ideas include the following:

- First Responders must keep their practice within the scope of care as defined by the state.

- Among a First Responder's ethical responsibilities is to serve the physical and emotional needs of the patient with respect for human dignity and with no regard to nationality, race, gender, creed, or status.

- Before providing emergency care to any patient, you must determine the patient's competence and get either expressed or implied consent.

- A competent adult has the right to refuse treatment or to withdraw from treatment for him- or herself or for his or her child. Follow state law and local protocols in regard to advance directives.

- As a First Responder, you have a duty to act, or a legal obligation to provide care to a patient who needs it and consents to it. If there is a breach of duty, you could be charged with abandonment or negligence.

- A patient's history, condition, and emergency care are confidential. You must have a written form signed by the patient or legal guardian before you can release this information, unless you are required by law to share it.

- When you are called to a potential crime scene, the police must be notified. Do not enter a crime scene until it has been secured by the police and they tell you it is safe to do so. Once on scene, your priority is patient care. However, take all necessary precautions to preserve any potential evidence.

- Special reporting situations in your state may include reporting child, elderly, or spouse abuse; injury that is the result of a crime including sexual assault; and infectious disease exposure.

CONTENT REVIEW

▼

1. As a First Responder, you are allowed to perform only certain defined skills. These skills are called your:
   a. duty to act.
   b. scope of care.
   c. standard of care.
   d. ethical responsibilities.

2. List six of a First Responder's ethical responsibilities.

   a.

   b.

   c.

   d.

   e.

   f.

3. A competent adult is one who is:
   a. any person over the age of 18 or 21.
   b. lucid and able to make an informed decision.
   c. married, a parent, or a member of the armed forces.
   d. seriously ill or injured, which could affect judgment.

4. In order for consent to be valid, the patient must be _____ and the consent must be _____ .
   a. alert, understood
   b. informed, written
   c. competent, informed
   d. persuaded, expressed

5. Expressed consent may be any of the following EXCEPT:
   a. oral.
   b. a nod.
   c. implied.
   d. an affirming gesture.

6. Whose responsibility is it to make sure the patient understands the First Responder's plan for emergency care, including the risks?
   a. the First Responder
   b. the patient's lawyer
   c. the patient's physician
   d. the EMS medical director

7. As a First Responder, how might you go about getting a responsive, competent adult's expressed consent?

8. An example of an advance directive is a(n):
   a. emancipated minor.
   b. prehospital care report.
   c. refusal-of-treatment form.
   d. living will or DNR order.

9. You arrive at a scene where you find a 22-year-old woman who has apparently overdosed on heroin. She is unresponsive. You begin to initiate treatment based on the idea of _____ consent.
   a. actual
   b. substituted
   c. implied
   d. mandatory

10. You are at the scene of a terminally ill patient who has gone into respiratory arrest in your presence. The patient's daughter arrives on scene and insists that you withhold treatment. How should you proceed? Explain your answer.

11. If a First Responder forces care on a patient who refuses it, the First Responder may be charged with:
    a. assault and battery.
    b. abandonment and assault.
    c. battery and attempted rape.
    d. negligence and breach of duty.

12. List six actions you should take before leaving the scene of a moderately injured adult patient who has refused your treatment.

    a.

    b.

    c.

    d.

    e.

    f.

13. The term _____ is defined as terminating care of a patient without making sure that care will continue at the same level or higher.
    a. negligence
    b. abandonment
    c. assault
    d. battery

14. If a First Responder's care deviates from the accepted standard of care and results in further injury to the patient, the First Responder may be guilty of:
    a. negligence.
    b. abandonment.
    c. assault.
    d. battery.

15. A medical identification tag is meant to inform health care workers of:
    a. the preference for private over public hospitals.
    b. physical characteristics such as a limp or stutter.
    c. a medical condition such as an allergy or diabetes.
    d. the patient's medical insurance company ID number.

16. A First Responder with the fire department arrives on scene just in time to see a woman being carried away from a fire to safety. The woman's clothes are still smoldering. Very quickly, the First Responder realizes this patient needs more help than he can provide. Does the First Responder have a duty to act? Explain your answer.

17. Jake works in a factory on an assembly line. He is also one of three employees who were trained as on-site First Responders. One day on the way to work, Jake spots a car crash along the highway. Does he have a duty to act? Explain your answer.

18. In general, _____ includes the patient's history, condition, and emergency care.
    a. assault and battery
    b. preservation of evidence
    c. confidential information
    d. the public's right to know

19. Under "Good Samaritan" laws, a person suing an emergency care provider must prove that the emergency care was markedly below the:
    a. duty to act.
    b. standard of care.
    c. reasonable standard.
    d. negligence threshold.

20. The term "standard of care" refers to the care that would be expected to be provided to the same patient under the same conditions:
    a. according to the Hippocratic oath.
    b. before taking care of other patients.
    c. in a fair, reasonable, and unbiased way.
    d. by another First Responder who has the same training.

21. You are responding to a crime scene. Which of the following rules of thumb is NOT true?
    a. If the crime is in progress, do not try to provide care.
    b. As you provide emergency care, try to preserve all possible evidence.
    c. Patient confidentiality forbids you from reporting an injury that may have resulted from a crime.
    d. You may be required to report injuries from suspected child abuse.

22. List three examples of emergencies you may be legally required to report to law enforcement or another appropriate authority or agency.

    a.

    b.

    c.

CASE STUDY: THE PATIENT
WHO WILL NOT GO TO THE HOSPITAL

▼

Read this scenario and answer the questions that follow. Focus on the rights that adult patients have regarding consent to medical care, as well as the obligation of First Responders to encourage patients to go to the hospital should they appear to need medical care.

It is two o'clock in the morning. You are working on the engine at your volunteer fire department when you are paged out to respond to a possible heart attack. You arrive to find an elderly patient, Mr. Boyd, sitting on the edge of his bed. During your initial assessment, you notice that he appears to be slightly sweaty and pale. He tells you that he had a bout of chest pain that felt the same as the heart attack he had one year ago. He took three of his nitroglycerin pills, which relieved the pain. He says he is feeling much better and does not wish to go to the emergency room. The paramedic ambulance, which is coming from the next town, has yet to arrive. His wife says he really needs to be taken to the emergency room and that his last heart attack "almost killed him."

23. Does this patient need to go to the hospital? Explain your answer.

24. Describe two strategies you might use to convince the patient that he should go with the paramedics to the hospital.

    a.

    b.

Mr. Boyd is still refusing treatment and transport even after the paramedics arrive and complete their assessment. By now his skin has dried and he appears less pale. He states that he is pain-free, has no other symptoms, and that he will follow up with his doctor in the morning. His vital signs appear stable, and he is fully alert. The paramedics have by now become frustrated with Mr. Boyd's reluctance to go to the emergency room with them. In exasperation, they tell him that if he will not go voluntarily, they will force him to go against his will. A wrestling match ensues, with Mr. Boyd finally restrained on a wheeled stretcher.

25. Do you agree with the paramedics' strategy? What rights does an alert adult patient have to refuse treatment and transport?

CHAPTER 4

THE HUMAN BODY

KEY IDEAS
▼

This chapter introduces you to basic anatomy and physiology. Key ideas include the following:

- An understanding of key anatomical and topographic terms is important for describing a patient's position, as well as the location of injuries and other physical findings.

- The body is divided into three main cavities: thoracic, abdominal, and pelvic.

- Major body systems are the skeletal, muscular, circulatory, respiratory, digestive, urinary, endocrine, reproductive, nervous, and integument (skin) systems.

- Understanding the anatomy and physiology of these systems is critical if you are to understand your patients' injuries and illnesses.

CONTENT REVIEW
▼

1. Match the following terms of position to their correct descriptions.

    anatomical •   • face up, lying on the back

    lateral recumbent •   • face down, lying on the stomach

    prone •   • standing, arms down, palms out

    supine •   • lying on the side

2. The injury to the patient's abdomen was _____ to the bottom of the sternum.
    a. inferior
    b. superior
    c. anterior
    d. posterior

3. The _____ thorax includes the chest and abdomen.
    a. inferior
    b. superior
    c. anterior
    d. posterior

4. The patient suffered a _____ injury, which was less than an eighth of an inch deep.
   a. deep
   b. medial
   c. lateral
   d. superficial

5. The entrance wound from the bullet was _____ to the left nipple. It almost looked as though it had entered through the patient's left side.
   a. deep
   b. medial
   c. lateral
   d. superficial

6. The bruise to the patient's chest was _____ to the right nipple, along the right border of the sternum.
   a. deep
   b. medial
   c. lateral
   d. superficial

7. The patient was experiencing _____ neck pain where the back of her neck impacted the headrest during a collision.
   a. posterior
   b. anterior
   c. proximal
   d. distal

8. The fracture to the patient's leg appeared to be to the lower thigh, just _____ to the knee.
   a. posterior
   b. anterior
   c. proximal
   d. distal

9. The patient had a forearm fracture. She was able to feel a strong pulse _____ to the injury, at the patient's wrist.
   a. posterior
   b. anterior
   c. proximal
   d. distal

10. The swelling to the patient's face was isolated to the cheek, just _____ to the left eye.
   a. inferior
   b. superior
   c. anterior
   d. posterior

11. Complete the puzzle.

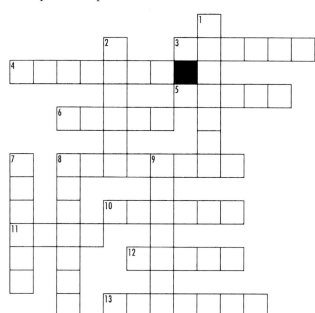

ACROSS

3. A bone of the forearm
4. Shoulder blade
5. A bone of the upper leg
6. Eye socket
8. _____ spine, or neck
10. Part of the spine formed by five fused vertebrae
11. A bone of the forearm
12. A bone of the lower leg
13. A bone of the upper arm

DOWN

1. Knee cap
2. The lower back
7. A bone of the lower leg
8. Bones that form top, back, and sides of skull
9. Hip bone

12. The abdominal cavity is separated from the thoracic cavity by the:
    a. ribs.
    b. lungs.
    c. stomach.
    d. diaphragm.

13. The lungs and heart are found in the _____ cavity.
    a. pelvic
    b. cranial
    c. thoracic
    d. abdominal

14. The intestines are found in the _____ cavity.
    a. pelvic
    b. cranial
    c. thoracic
    d. abdominal

15. The _____ cavity is bounded by the lower part of the spine, hip bones, and pubis.
    a. pelvic
    b. cranial
    c. thoracic
    d. abdominal

16. The largest part of the liver is located in the _____ quadrant of the abdomen.
    a. left upper
    b. left lower
    c. right upper
    d. right lower

17. The left kidney is located in the _____ quadrant of the abdomen.
    a. left upper
    b. left lower
    c. right upper
    d. right lower

18. The spleen is located in the _____ quadrant of the abdomen.
    a. left upper
    b. left lower
    c. right upper
    d. right lower

19. Ligaments connect:
    a. bone to bone.
    b. muscle to bone.
    c. different layers of muscle.
    d. internal organs to bone and muscle.

20. The side impact from the car crash broke the patient's upper arm, or:
    a. ulna.
    b. radius.
    c. humerus.
    d. patella.

21. The _____ is made up of the top, back, and sides of the skull.
    a. femur
    b. cranium
    c. mandible
    d. iliac crest

22. The _____ is made up of 33 bones called vertebrae.
    a. coccyx
    b. lumbar spine
    c. spinal column
    d. xiphoid process

23. The bones that make up the shoulder girdle are the:
    a. clavicle and scapula.
    b. humerus and radius.
    c. ileum and ischium.
    d. tibia and fibula.

24. Explain the difference between smooth and skeletal muscles.

25. The passage of air into and out of the lungs is called:
    a. exhalation.
    b. expiration.
    c. respiration.
    d. inspiration.

26. All of the following are related to breathing and the respiratory system EXCEPT:
    a. alveoli.
    b. bronchi.
    c. larynx.
    d. pharynx.
    e. trachea.
    f. ventricle.
    g. epiglottis.
    h. oropharynx.
    i. bronchiole.
    j. nasopharynx.

27. The area posterior to the mouth and nose is called the:
    a. pharynx.
    b. diaphragm.
    c. costal cartilage.
    d. left main bronchus.

28. After air enters the mouth and nose, it passes through the _____ , down through the _____ , and into the _____ .
    a. pharynx, larynx, trachea.
    b. trachea, larynx, pharynx.
    c. pharynx, nasopharynx, oropharynx.
    d. oropharynx, nasopharynx, pharynx.

29. Use words from the list below to complete the sentences. Note that not all the words in the list are used and some may be used more than once.

    smaller   harder   more
    larger   softer   less

    a. Every part of an infant or child's airway is _____ than an adult's.

    b. In children the tongue takes up _____ space than an adult's.

    c. In infants the tongue is _____ likely to cause a blocked airway.

    d. The trachea of an infant or child is _____ flexible, narrower, and

       _____ than the trachea of an adult.

30. The smallest vessels through which the exchange of fluid, oxygen, and carbon dioxide takes place are called:
    a. alveoli.
    b. venules.
    c. arterioles.
    d. capillaries.

31. Draw a line to connect each arterial pulse point to its correct location.

carotid •   • upper arm

femoral •   • wrist

brachial •   • thigh

radial •   • foot

dorsal pedis •   • neck

32. The organs of the digestive system include all of the following EXCEPT:
    a. pancreas.
    b. epidermis.
    c. esophagus.
    d. alimentary tract.

33. Which system consists of two kidneys, two ureters, one urinary bladder, and one urethra?
    a. urinary
    b. endocrine
    c. digestive
    d. reproductive

34. Which of the following is NOT true of the endocrine system?
    a. It influences behavior.
    b. It stimulates breathing.
    c. It influences reproduction.
    d. It affects physical strength.

35. Which system includes ovaries and fallopian tubes?
    a. urinary
    b. endocrine
    c. digestive
    d. reproductive

CASE STUDY: ANATOMY AND PHYSIOLOGY APPLIED

▼

Read the scenario below and answer the questions that follow. Focus on how knowledge of anatomy and physiology can help you to manage patients in the field.

You have just responded to an unhelmeted bicyclist who was hit by a car and thrown onto the pavement. She is complaining of pain to the upper right quadrant of her abdomen and to her right chest. She has suffered huge scrapes to her side and abdomen. She has a large bruise on her forehead. In addition, she does not remember the accident and continues to repeat the same confused questions over and over. Her breathing appears rapid and labored.

36. Which abdominal organs may be injured?

37. An injury to which system is probably causing this patient to be confused?

38. Her rapid breathing is quite noticeable. It is obvious to you that this patient has a problem with her respiratory system. Would you treat this problem before or after treating her abdominal pain and scrapes to her skin? Explain your answer.

39. You examine the patient further and find that she has a leg injury. It appears that the large bone of her lower leg is fractured just below the knee. The fracture has caused the lower leg to be turned away from the midline of her body. Using the terms described on pages 43–44 of your text, describe the position of the leg and its injuries.

CHAPTER 5

LIFTING AND MOVING PATIENTS

KEY IDEAS

This chapter provides an overview of how to lift and move patients and equipment safely, without injury to the patients and without injury to you. Key ideas include the following:

- Incorrect lifting and handling of patients can worsen their injuries and cause career-ending injuries to rescuers.

- There may be instances in which you must move a patient prior to treating him or her due to hazards, inaccessibility, or other problems.

- Emergency techniques for moving patients include the shirt drag, blanket drag, and shoulder or forearm drag.

- Non-emergency, or non-urgent, moves include the direct ground lift and extremity lift.

- Equipment First Responders should be acquainted with and know how to use properly include standard stretchers, the stair chair, and backboards.

CONTENT REVIEW

▼

1. The term "body mechanics" refers to methods of:
   a. exercising to strengthen your back muscles.
   b. positioning the patient for safe extrication.
   c. using your body to gain a mechanical advantage.
   d. determining how a patient may have been injured.

2. List four basic safety rules of lifting any object.

   a.

   b.

   c.

   d.

3. Always try to reach _____ to lift a heavy object.
   a. up, not down
   b. a long distance
   c. a short distance
   d. with a power grip

4. The key to preventing injury during lifting, carrying, moving, reaching, pushing, and pulling is:
   a. correct alignment of your spine.
   b. balance, strength, and attitude.
   c. to keep your knees slightly bent.
   d. to lock your elbows, wrists, and knees.

5. In a power lift, you should _____ to splint your vulnerable lower back area.
   a. avoid excessive slouch or swayback
   b. take a long deep breath and hold it
   c. relax the muscles of your legs and buttocks
   d. tighten the muscles of your back and abdomen

6. Which one of the following describes good posture while standing?
   a. Knees are locked and pelvis is tucked back.
   b. Chin points out and shoulders are rolled forward.
   c. Chin, sternum, and knees are in vertical alignment.
   d. Ears, shoulders, and hips are in vertical alignment.

7. Which one of the following describes good posture while sitting?
   a. Knees are locked and pelvis is tucked back.
   b. Chin points out and shoulders are rolled forward.
   c. Chin, sternum, and knees are in vertical alignment.
   d. Ears, shoulders, and hips are in vertical alignment.

8. Identify all the items below that contribute to a balanced physical fitness program.

_____ a. cardiovascular conditioning

_____ b. flexibility training

_____ c. strength training

_____ d. good nutrition

9. Even when there is no immediate threat to life, you should move your patient to an area that is suited to the administration of emergency medical care.

_____ True

_____ False

10. List five conditions under which you would consider making an emergency move of your patient.

a.

b.

c.

d.

e.

11. The greatest danger to the patient during an emergency move is the possibility of making a spine injury worse.

_____ True

_____ False

12. Below are the steps a rescuer must take to perform a "forearm drag." Number the following steps 1–5 to show the order in which they should be performed.

_____ Drag the patient toward you.

_____ Stand at the patient's head.

_____ Grasp the patient's forearms.

_____ Slip your hands under the patient's armpits.

_____ Support the patient's head on your own forearms.

13. Rescuers should use an "extremity lift" when the patient has injuries to his or her arms or legs.

_____ True

_____ False

Questions 14, 15, and 16 may have more than one correct answer. Circle the letters next to all statements that seem correct for each question.

14. Pole stretchers are usually used when there:
   a. are multiple patients.
   b. are flights of stairs to navigate.
   c. is not enough space for a standard stretcher.
   d. is a spinal injury accompanied by unresponsiveness.

15. What type of stretcher can be used to lift a patient from a confined area where a larger stretcher will not fit?
   a. stair chair
   b. scoop stretcher
   c. standard stretcher with wheeled legs
   d. vest-type immobilization device

16. Which of the following pieces of equipment should be used for moving a patient with a possible spinal injury?
   a. backboard
   b. stair chair
   c. pole stretcher
   d. blanket stretcher

17. What kinds of materials can be used to improvise a stretcher?

CASE STUDY:
TO MOVE OR NOT TO MOVE

▼

Read this scenario and answer the questions that follow. Focus on when you may need to move patients.

Your unit has been staged at the local high school during a football game. It is almost the end of the first half when spectators start screaming. A section of the old bleachers has collapsed, trapping five people.

18. What are your first responsibilities? Name at least two.

19. Along with school authorities, you are able to move the crowd of spectators away from the collapsed structure, leaving only those trapped at the scene. What would you need to consider in order to make an emergency move of these patients?

20. Decide if you would move each patient described below right away. Write the reason for your answer.

   a. Patient #1 is sitting at the edge of the collapsed structure with a board over her legs. She is complaining only of knee pain and reports that she fell straight down about two feet onto her buttocks.

   b. Patients #2 and #3 are on top of patient #4. Patients #2 and #3 are awake and complaining of leg and arm pain. They are scared because they cannot wake up patient #4 and cannot feel him breathing.

   c. Patient #5 is trapped in some metal debris. He says that he cannot move his legs and that his neck hurts. There are no other dangers around him.

CHAPTER 6

AIRWAY

KEY IDEAS
▼

Airway and breathing management are the most important tasks performed by First Responders. Key ideas include the following:

- The first priority in any emergency is to establish and maintain a patient's airway. Without an open airway or adequate respirations, a patient will die within minutes.

- Accurate and efficient patient assessment will provide you with the information you need to determine whether or not your patient requires airway or breathing assistance.

- A patient's airway may need to be opened using either the head-tilt/chin-lift or the jaw-thrust maneuver.

- Breathing is assessed using the look, listen, and feel method.

- Artificial ventilation, or rescue breathing, is the procedure used to ventilate patients who are not breathing or who are breathing inadequately.

- First Responders must learn to assess and treat patients with both partial and complete airway obstructions. Different methods are used for treating infant, child, and adult patients.

- Aids to resuscitation also can be used to help patients with airway or breathing problems. They include airway adjuncts such as oral and nasal airways, suction units, oxygen-administration equipment, and bag-valve-mask devices.

CONTENT REVIEW

1. Trace the flow of air through the respiratory tract during inhalation. Number the following items 1–6 in the correct sequence.

    _____ alveoli

    _____ pharynx

    _____ mouth and nose

    _____ trachea

    _____ bronchial tubes

    _____ larynx

2. Circle the letter next to the item(s) that describe what happens during inhalation.
    a. The patient's rib muscles contract.
    b. Air pressure inside the lungs decreases.
    c. The patient's diaphragm falls and flattens.
    d. Air pressure inside the lungs is increased.

3. Circle the letter next to the item(s) that describe what happens during exhalation.
    a. The patient's diaphragm rises.
    b. The patient's chest muscles relax.
    c. Air pressure inside the lungs decreases.
    d. Air pressure inside the lungs increases.

4. Fill in the missing information from the table below.

	Normal Breathing Rates
Adult	_____ to _____ breaths per minute
Child	_____ to _____ breaths per minute
Infant	_____ to _____ breaths per minute

5. The chest wall is softer in infants than in adults. So _____ can alert you to respiratory distress in an infant.
    a. the epiglottis
    b. excessive movement
    c. wheezing and stridor
    d. air pressure inside the chest

6. Why can tipping an infant's head back or allowing the head to fall forward be a problem?
    a. It will make breathing effortless.
    b. The positions can close the trachea.
    c. The diaphragm will fall and flatten.
    d. Because the chest wall is softer in infants.

7. The tongue of an infant or child takes up more space than in an adult. It therefore can:
   a. use a back blow immediately.
   b. block the airway more easily.
   c. keep the trachea open more often.
   d. loosen the cricoid cartilage quickly.

8. When you perform a head-tilt/chin-lift on an infant or child, you should:
   a. hyperextend only the head.
   b. hyperextend the head and neck.
   c. tilt the head back only slightly.
   d. tilt the head back as far as possible.

9. Describe how to perform a head-tilt/chin-lift maneuver on an adult patient.

10. The head-tilt/chin-lift and jaw-thrust maneuvers:
    a. align the nasal passages with the throat.
    b. align the pharynx with the epiglottis.
    c. lift the tongue away from the throat.
    d. flex the windpipe at a 90° angle.

11. Your patient fell six feet onto concrete from a ladder. Which of the following methods would you use to open her airway?
    a. recovery position
    b. jaw-thrust maneuver
    c. head-neck/in-line move
    d. head-tilt/chin-lift maneuver

12. You are at the scene of a patient who was found unresponsive in his bed. His wife insists that there has been no fall or other blow that may have caused a recent injury. To open the patient's airway, use a:
    a. recovery position.
    b. jaw-thrust maneuver.
    c. head-neck/in-line move.
    d. head-tilt/chin-lift maneuver.

13. The oropharyngeal airway is used to maintain the airway of an unresponsive patient who has a gag reflex.

_____ True

_____ False

14. To determine the proper size oropharyngeal airway for your patient, measure it from the:
    a. lips to the base of the tongue.
    b. corner of the nose to the top of the ear.
    c. tip of the nose to the tip of the earlobe.
    d. corner of the lip to the angle of the jaw.

15. Briefly describe how to insert an oropharyngeal airway in an adult patient.

16. To use an oropharyngeal airway in an infant or child, insert it:
    a. tip side up.
    b. flange side first.
    c. in its upright position.
    d. in an upside-down position.

17. The nasopharyngeal airway is used to maintain the airway of a patient who has a gag reflex.

_____ True

_____ False

18. To determine the proper size nasopharyngeal airway for your patient, measure it from the:
    a. lips to the base of the tongue.
    b. corner of the nose to the top of the ear.
    c. tip of the nose to the tip of the earlobe.
    d. corner of the lip to the angle of the jaw.

19. Briefly describe how to insert a nasopharyngeal airway in an adult patient.

20. If during insertion of a nasopharyngeal airway you meet resistance, you should try:
a. finger sweeps and suctioning.
b. an oropharyngeal airway instead.
c. inserting it from the other end.
d. inserting it into the other nostril.

21. You have just inserted a nasopharyngeal airway into your patient's nostril. As you reassess the patient's condition, you find that he is breathing spontaneously but you can detect no air movement through the tube. What should you do?
a. Remove the adjunct airway immediately.
b. Insert an oropharyngeal airway immediately.
c. Place the patient in the recovery position.
d. Rotate the adjunct airway from side to side.

22. To help maintain an open airway in an unresponsive patient who has not been injured, is breathing adequately, and has a pulse:
a. insert an airway adjunct.
b. suspect gastric distention.
c. place him or her in a recovery position.
d. perform a finger sweep and suction.

23. Describe the procedure for using a suctioning device. Number the following items 1–5 in the correct sequence.

_____ Take BSI precautions.

_____ Turn on the suction unit.

_____ Apply the suction catheter from side to side.

_____ Insert the catheter to the base of the tongue.

_____ Select the correct type catheter for your patient.

24. Use suctioning for up to _____ second(s) in an infant, _____ seconds for a child, and _____ seconds for an adult.
a. 2, 2, 2
b. 3, 6, 9
c. 5, 10, 15
d. 7, 13, 21

25. Briefly describe in three steps how you can determine the presence of breathing in your patient.

a.

b.

c.

26. An ominous sign of inadequate breathing is a slower than normal breathing rate. Fill in the table below.

	Inadequate Breathing
Adult	Less than _____ respirations per minute
Child	Less than _____ respirations per minute
Infant	Less than _____ respirations per minute

27. Circle the letters next to the signs and symptoms of inadequate breathing.
   a. Drowsiness, confusion
   b. Flaring of the nostrils
   c. Increased effort to breathe
   d. Inadequate chest wall motion
   e. Seesaw motion of abdomen and chest
   f. 18 breaths per minute in an infant
   g. 15 breaths per minute in a child
   h. 12 breaths per minute in an adult
   i. Gasping and grunting sounds with breathing
   j. Unequal rise and fall of the sides of the chest
   k. Slow heart rate accompanied by slow breathing rate
   l. Retractions between the ribs or above the collarbone
   m. Bluish discoloration of the skin or mucous membranes

28. Briefly describe four indications of adequate ventilations.

   a.

   b.

   c.

   d.

29. Briefly describe three indications of inadequate ventilations.

   a.

   b.

   c.

30. Mouth-to-mask ventilation is preferred over the mouth-to-mouth and mouth-to-barrier device techniques. Circle the letters beside the reasons why.
   a. It frees your hands for other emergency care needs.
   b. It eliminates exposure to the patient's exhaled air.
   c. It allows you to deliver ventilations of adequate force.
   d. It prevents direct contact with a patient's body fluids.

31. You must maintain a jaw-thrust maneuver during artificial ventilation of a patient with suspected spinal injury.

_____ True

_____ False

32. List the basic steps of mouth-to-mask ventilation.

33. Fill in the missing information from the table below.

	Artificial Ventilation Rates
Adult	_____ breaths per minute at _____ to _____ seconds each.
Child	_____ breaths per minute at _____ to _____ seconds each.
Infant	_____ breaths per minute at _____ to _____ seconds each.
Newborn	_____ breaths per minute at _____ to _____ seconds each.

34. You attempt to ventilate an unresponsive patient for the first time and find that you are unable to force air into the lungs. Your next step should be to:
   a. check for a foreign body airway obstruction.
   b. reposition the patient's head and try again.
   c. suction the patient's airway for 15 seconds.
   d. insert a nasopharyngeal airway and try again.

35. A patient who has had all or part of the larynx surgically removed has had a:
   a. thoracostomy
   b. tracheostomy.
   c. pneumonectomy.
   d. laryngectomy.

36. A _____ is a permanent opening that connects the trachea directly to the front of the neck.
    a. stoma
    b. larynx
    c. stamen
    d. stollen

37. You are at the scene of a near-drowning of a 10-month-old baby. The patient has a pulse but is not breathing. Your crew members are inexperienced at managing such a young patient, and they need your help. Respond to the following concerns.

    a. "How should we open this kid's airway? Same as an adult's?"

    b. "I'm having a really hard time fitting my mouth around the baby's mouth. It's so small. What should I do?"

    c. "How often should I breathe for this kid?"

38. Which of the following is NOT a recommended method for reducing gastric distention in an infant or child?
    a. Gently press down on the patient's abdomen.
    b. Breathe slowly when ventilating the patient.
    c. Avoid ventilating the patient too forcefully.
    d. Allow the patient to fully exhale between ventilations.

39. To provide artificial ventilation by way of a bag-valve-mask device, one rescuer should

    _____ while the other _____

    until the patient's chest rises.

40. Patients require supplemental oxygen if they have any condition that prevents an efficient flow of oxygen throughout their bodies. List three of these conditions.

a.

b.

c.

41. The following list includes safety precautions you should take when you handle oxygen cylinders. Circle the letters next to the statements that are true:
a. Never store cylinders below 125°F.
b. Never "crack" a tank with a wrench.
c. Never allow smoking near an oxygen cylinder.
d. Never place your body over the cylinder valve.
e. Always stand a cylinder upright near a patient.
f. Always keep cylinder valves closed when not in use.
g. Keep cylinders secured, especially during transport.
h. All cylinders must have the correct regulator valves.
i. Never allow combustible materials to touch the cylinder.

42. Describe how to administer oxygen to a patient. Number the following steps 1–9 in the correct sequence.

___2___ Remove the protective seal.

___1___ Identify the cylinder as oxygen.

___4___ Position the regulator and align the pins.

___5___ Hand-tighten the T-screw on the regulator.

___8___ Adjust the flow meter to the proper liter flow.

___9___ Apply the oxygen delivery device to the patient.

___3___ Crack the main cylinder to remove dust and debris.

___7___ Attach the oxygen delivery device to the regulator.

___6___ Open the main cylinder valve and check the pressure.

43. An oxygen delivery device that provides up to 90% oxygen and is made up of a reservoir bag and a one-way valve is a:
a. nasal cannula.
b. airway adjunct.
c. pocket face mask.
d. nonrebreather mask.

44. An oxygen delivery device that provides up to 44% oxygen and is good for patients who are anxious about a mask and patients who are nauseated or vomiting is a:
   a. nasal cannula.
   b. airway adjunct.
   c. pocket face mask.
   d. nonrebreather mask.

45. The most common cause of an airway obstruction in an unresponsive patient is:
   a. food.
   b. dentures.
   c. the tongue.
   d. aspirated vomit.

46. The treatment for a partial airway obstruction in an adult with good air exchange includes:
   a. encouraging the patient to cough up the foreign body.
   b. delivering five back blows for each abdominal thrust.
   c. having the patient get into a supine position.
   d. dislodging the object with finger sweeps.

47. When relieving a complete airway obstruction in a responsive adult patient, you should alternate back blows with abdominal thrusts.

   _____ True

   _____ False

48. Describe the four basic steps for clearing a foreign body airway obstruction in a responsive adult.

   a.

   b.

   c.

   d.

49. You are managing a 17-year-old patient with an airway obstruction. After you apply several abdominal thrusts, the patient falls to the ground unconscious. What should you do next?
   a. Perform five more abdominal thrusts.
   b. Attempt chest thrusts as you would for CPR.
   c. Place the patient in the recovery position.
   d. Perform a tongue-jaw lift and a finger sweep.

50. All of the following patients have a foreign body airway obstruction. Which one(s) should receive the recommended treatment for an adult?
    a. one-year-old
    b. three-year-old
    c. five-year-old
    d. seven-year-old
    e. nine-year-old
    f. eleven-year-old
    g. thirteen-year-old

51. Suspect an infection in an infant who has sudden onset of respiratory distress with coughing, gagging, stridor, or wheezing, especially when food or small items are found near the patient.

    _____ True

    _____ False

52. An eight-month-old baby has a partial foreign body airway obstruction with poor air exchange. You may attempt to relieve the obstruction with back blows and chest thrusts.

    _____ True

    _____ False

53. After you determine that you must relieve a foreign body airway obstruction in an infant, you should proceed as follows. (Write the numerals 1–6 to show the correct sequence of steps.)

    __2__ Deliver up to five back blows.

    __5__ Deliver up to five chest thrusts.

    __4__ Position your hand on the infant's sternum.

    __3__ Turn the infant face up, with head lower than body.

    __1__ Straddle the infant face down over one of your arms.

    __6__ Alternate sets of blows and thrusts until object is expelled.

54. If you are alone, and you are unable to open the airway of an infant who is found unresponsive, you must activate the EMS system within:
    a. 15 seconds.
    b. 30 seconds.
    c. 1 minute.
    d. 3 minutes.

55. Your patient is an infant with a foreign body airway obstruction who is found unresponsive. Write the numerals 1–6 to describe the correct sequence of steps you should take.

___2___ Deliver five back blows.

___3___ Deliver five chest thrusts.

___4___ Perform a tongue-jaw lift.

___1___ Open the airway, and deliver breaths.

___5___ If you see the object, perform a finger sweep.

___6___ If the obstruction is not relieved, repeat the procedure.

CASE STUDY: A DROWNING VICTIM

▼

Read this scenario and answer the questions that follow. Focus on correctly assessing the patient's airway and breathing status and arriving at the appropriate airway and ventilation interventions. Watch the patient for status changes.

It is early afternoon on a hot summer day, and you are dispatched to the call that you have always dreaded: a pediatric drowning. You arrive on scene—a suburban residence, gather your equipment, and run around to the backyard pool. There you are greeted by three adults. They are crowded around the limp body of a two-year-old, who is lying by the side of the pool. They are screaming and crying and frantically yelling at you to hurry. As you approach the child, named Gracie, you learn that she fell into the pool without striking her head, neck, or back. She lay submerged for one or two minutes before being pulled out of the water by her mother.

You move to Gracie's side and note that she is unresponsive and blue. Gracie's mother is nearly sitting on top of you as she screams and cries. Your partner, John, shouts something to you as he approaches, but you are unable to hear him over the din.

56. What should be your first action in this situation?

57. One of the adults yells at you, "Do something! You need to breathe for her! She's not breathing!" Do you agree that this should be your first step? Explain your answer.

58. You determine that you need to breathe for Gracie. Number the following actions 1–3 to place the steps in the correct order.

_____3_____ **a.** Continue ventilations at a rate of 20 breaths per minute.

_____1_____ **b.** Deliver two slow initial breaths.

_____2_____ **c.** Determine if the ventilations are adequate.

59. Gracie's stomach appears to have gotten slightly distended. What steps can you take to stop this problem from continuing?

60. Gracie suddenly vomits. What should you do?

61. After ventilating Gracie for two to three minutes, you notice that her color is improving dramatically. She begins moving her limbs, and her eyelids begin to flutter and twitch. Your next step should be to:

CHAPTER 7

CIRCULATION

KEY IDEAS

Heart disease kills many Americans each year. Patients who are in cardiac arrest require immediate CPR and early advanced care if they are to have any chance of surviving. This chapter focuses on recognizing patients in cardiac arrest and correctly applying CPR. Key ideas include the following:

- Patients in cardiac arrest need immediate CPR followed by advanced medical care, including defibrillation (shocking the heart) within eight to ten minutes.

- CPR helps to oxygenate and circulate the blood until advanced care can be given. Any delay in performing CPR reduces the chance that the patient will survive.

- Before providing CPR to your patient, you must first establish unresponsiveness, breathlessness, and pulselessness.

- The EMS system should be activated as soon as you determine an adult patient is unresponsive. For infants and children, activate EMS after one minute of basic life support.

- CPR may be performed by either one or two rescuers.

- You may stop CPR only if you are exhausted and unable to continue, if you have turned your patient over to another trained rescuer or the hospital staff, if the patient is resuscitated, or if the patient has been declared dead by a proper authority.

CONTENT REVIEW

▼

1. Which statement(s) below are true about the heart?
   a. The left side receives oxygenated blood from the lungs.
   b. The right side receives oxygenated blood from the lungs.
   c. The left side pumps blood to the lungs to be oxygenated.
   d. The right side pumps blood to the lungs to be oxygenated.

2. Which statement(s) below are true about an adult patient's pulse?
   a. It is a sign of the pressure exerted by each contraction of the heart.
   b. The waves of blood the heart sends to the body are felt as the pulse.
   c. It is felt where a large artery lies over a bone close to the skin.
   d. At rest an adult's should be between 60 and 80 beats per minute.

3. Which statement(s) below are true about clinical death?
   a. After 4 to 6 minutes brain cells begin to die.
   b. Immediate CPR and advanced care cannot reverse it.
   c. It occurs when a patient is breathless and pulseless.
   d. After 8 to 10 minutes irreversible damage occurs to the brain.

4. The letters "CPR" stand for:
   a. cardiac pain relaxation.
   b. cardiographic radiation.
   c. cardiopulmonary resuscitation.
   d. cardiocompression ratification.

5. The "chain of survival" includes four links. List them.

   a.

   b.

   c.

   d.

6. List the four conditions under which CPR may be discontinued.

   a.

   b.

   c.

   d.

7. To determine pulselessness in an adult patient, assess the _____ pulse point.
   a. pedis
   b. radial
   c. brachial
   d. carotid

8. The following list should describe the steps preceding CPR of an adult patient. Fill in the steps that are missing.

   Step 1: Determine unresponsiveness.

   Step 2:

   Step 3: Position the patient on a firm, flat surface.

   Step 4:

   Step 5:

   Step 6: Perform artificial ventilation.

   Step 7:

   Step 8: Begin CPR.

9. For you to properly perform CPR, the patient must be in a _____ position.
   a. prone
   b. supine
   c. recovery
   d. semi-sitting

10. To properly perform CPR, the patient must be on a _____ surface.
    a. hard flat
    b. soft flat
    c. soft tilted
    d. hard tilted

11. Before you may begin chest compressions, you always must determine that your patient is:

    a.

    b.

    c.

12. You will perform one-rescuer CPR on the following patients. Fill in the compression-to-breath ratio for each one.

    a. A 10-year-old:

    b. An 18-year-old:

    c. A 3-month-old:

    d. A 4-year-old:

13. You will perform one-rescuer CPR on the following patients. For each one, write in the correct hand description and position from the list.

heel of one hand   on lower half of sternum
two hands   on top third of sternum
two or three fingers   on top half of sternum

  a. A 5-month-old:

  b. A 7-year-old:

  c. A 71-year-old:

  d. A 36-year-old:

14. Fill in the chart below with the correct compression rate and depth for each patient.

	Infant	Child	Adult
Rate	_____ per minute	_____ per minute	_____ per minute
Depth	_____ to _____ inch(es)	_____ to _____ inch(es)	_____ to _____ inch(es)

15. Number the following actions 1–8 to correctly order the sequence of steps for adult CPR.

  _2_ Uncover your patient's chest.

  _3_ Get in position beside the patient.

  _6_ Thrust down and depress the sternum.

  _5_ Position your hands and your shoulders.

  _1_ Position the patient on a firm flat surface.

  _4_ Locate the xiphoid process and the compression site.

  _7_ Completely release pressure to allow blood to flow back into the heart.

16. You are observing another student practice adult CPR. You notice that one of your students is determining his hand position by placing the heel of one hand directly over the xiphoid process. He then places his other hand on top of this hand and begins compressions. Do you agree with this hand placement? Disagree? Explain your answer.

17. You observe another student using jerky, jabbing movements while performing chest compressions. You advise her that she needs to perform compressions more smoothly. She asks, "Why?" What is your answer?

18. Describe the differences between one- and two-person CPR by filling in the chart below.

	One-Rescuer CPR	Two-Rescuer CPR
Ratio of compressions to ventilations	_____ : _____	_____ : _____
Check pulse after:	_____ minute(s)	_____ minute(s)

19. Your class is reviewing the time rule for interrupting CPR. One of the students states, "CPR should only be stopped for five seconds." Is this always possible? Give your student an example of a time he or she may need to stop CPR for more than five seconds.

20. List three injuries that can occur when CPR is performed.

a.

b.

c.

21. To determine pulselessness in an infant, assess the _____ pulse point.
   a. pedis
   b. radial
   c. brachial
   d. carotid

22. To determine pulselessness in a child, assess the _____ pulse point.
   a. pedis
   b. radial
   c. brachial
   d. carotid

23. According to AHA guidelines, if you are alone, you must attempt to resuscitate an infant or child for three minutes before activating the EMS system.

_____ True

_____ False

24. The correct compression site for an infant is _____ an imaginary line between the nipples.
   a. one finger-width above
   b. one finger-width below
   c. two finger-widths above
   d. two finger-widths below

25. You have found Mr. Smith, a 65-year-old man, to be pulseless and breathless. When you begin compressions, you hear and feel a crunch. What should you do next? Why?

CASE STUDY: A CPR CALL

▼

Read this scenario and answer the questions that follow. Focus on the steps necessary to assess a patient and to provide CPR.

You and your partner are responding in the rescue unit to an "unknown medical." The dispatcher updates you with the information that a trained bystander is on scene and CPR has been started. You arrive at one of the local supermarkets and are led to a food aisle where the 70-year-old male patient has collapsed from an apparent heart attack. You find the bystander administering CPR amidst a pile of overturned canned goods, the patient's up-ended cart, and a pressing mass of onlookers.

26. What should your first action be?

27. If the person providing CPR needs to be relieved, what must you do?

28. But this person does not want to be relieved right away. So you observe. He is compressing the patient's chest with his hands placed on the patient's sternum in line with the patient's nipples. He is depressing the patient's chest about one inch at a rate of 60 compressions per minute. Critique his CPR method and offer suggestions, if necessary.

CHAPTER 8

AUTOMATED EXTERNAL DEFIBRILLATION

KEY IDEAS
▼

Early defibrillation is necessary to the cardiac-arrest patient's survival. In order to get it to the patient early enough, as many people as possible must be able to perform this life-saving skill. This chapter provides an overview. Key ideas include the following:

- Defibrillation by First Responders is indicated for an adult who is unresponsive, breathless, and pulseless.

- Defibrillation is the definitive treatment for certain heart rhythms. CPR maintains a patient until the defibrillator can be applied.

- The operator of an automated or semi-automated defibrillator must follow safety guidelines.

- Always treat the patient, not the machine. This means assessing the patient and also reassessing after each intervention, such as a shock or movement.

- Post-resuscitation care is needed to monitor return of pulses, make sure the patient is breathing, and note any changes in the patient's condition.

CONTENT REVIEW

1. What is defibrillation?

2. The letters "AED" stand for _____ defibrillation.
   a. automated external
   b. anatomical external
   c. automated electrical
   d. automatic electronic

3. A seven-year-old complained of her chest hurting and then collapsed. You have determined that she is unresponsive, breathless, and pulseless. Her airway is open. The paramedics will arrive in approximately two minutes. Should you start CPR or apply the AED? Why?

4. As your partner applies AED pads to the chest of an elderly woman, she tells him she is very afraid of the machine. He reassures her and tells her that her pulse is very slow and the AED will help her. He prevents everyone from touching the patient and presses the AED's "analyze" button. The machine advises a shock. Should this patient be shocked? Explain.

5. Could you use an AED on the following patients? Write "yes" or "no" beside each one.

   _____ a. A 12-year-old girl who weighs 85 pounds.

   _____ b. A 10-year-old boy who weighs 105 pounds.

   _____ c. A 32-year-old man who weighs 265 pounds.

   _____ d. A 14-year-old girl who weighs 112 pounds.

6. Explain why defibrillation should be attempted before CPR if the device is immediately available and responders trained in both AED use and CPR are present.

7. You are called to a cardiac-arrest patient with CPR in progress. When you arrive on scene with your AED ready to go, you find the patient is still unresponsive, breathless, and pulseless. Your next task is to:
   a. turn on the AED power.
   b. deliver a shock from the AED.
   c. apply the AED's adhesive pads to the patient.
   d. stop CPR and instruct everyone to clear the patient.

8. What should you do when the AED advises a shock? Number the following steps 1–8 to correctly order the steps.

   _____ Deliver the first shock.

   _____ Check the patient's pulse.

   _____ If you are advised, deliver a third shock.

   _____ If you are advised, deliver a second shock.

   _____ Wait until the AED reanalyzes the heart rhythm.

   _____ Wait until the AED reanalyzes the heart rhythm.

   _____ If there is no pulse, perform CPR for one minute.

9. Which of the following statements is correct?
   a. A non-working AED could be cause for legal action against your agency.
   b. AEDs need to be checked once a year according to the manufacturer's instructions.
   c. AEDs are simple devices and require no special care.
   d. AEDs only work after special drugs are given.

10. According to the AHA, defibrillation is a skill that:
    a. only physicians should be able to perform.
    b. requires a medical degree or its equivalent.
    c. all First Responders should be able to perform.
    d. anyone should perform, even without knowledge of CPR.

CASE STUDY: USING AN AED

▼

Read this scenario and answer the questions that follow. Focus on how to use an AED properly.

You and your partner are called to the corner store, where a middle-aged man was reported to have clutched his chest and slumped over in the seat of his car. Bystanders removed him to the ground and began CPR immediately.

After you arrive on scene and determine that it was safe to approach, you find two bystanders performing good CPR. Your partner assesses the patient while you set up the AED. The patient continues to be unresponsive, breathless, and pulseless.

11. When you open the patient's shirt, you find a nitroglycerin patch on the right upper chest wall. What should you do next?

12. You have attached the AED's adhesive pads to the patient's chest. The AED indicates that the patient should be shocked. What safety precaution should you take before pressing the "shock" button?

13. After the second shock is administered to your patient, the AED advises you to check the patient's pulse. You detect one. However, the patient is still breathless. What should you do now?

14. After three minutes of rescue breathing, your patient is breathing on his own at a rate of 20 times per minute. He has adequate chest rise, but he remains unresponsive without a gag reflex. At this point, what three things should you do?

    a.

    b.

    c.

CHAPTER 9

SCENE SIZE-UP

KEY IDEAS
▼

This chapter focuses on the safety of people on scene, identifying the mechanism of injury or nature of illness, and determining the necessary additional resources. Key ideas include the following:

- First Responders must ensure their own safety first. This involves planning, continued observation, and appropriate reaction to danger.

- Before entering the scene of an emergency, the First Responder must size it up for hazards and clues to the sequence of events.

- First Responders must use personal protective equipment appropriate to each call.

- Emergency medical care of a trauma patient depends on the pattern and extent of injury. The mechanism of injury can suggest what types of injuries occurred to the patient.

- It is part of scene size-up to determine and call for the appropriate resources needed on scene. Do this before you begin patient care.

1. Give two examples of how you can plan ahead to stay safe at an emergency scene.

   a.

   b.

2. Decide whether or not each of the following is a sign of danger at an emergency scene. If it is, give a reason why.

   a. You witness two people arguing.

   b. There is evidence of alcohol use.

   c. There is absolute silence.

3. When you find danger at an emergency scene, there are three actions you should take. They are:

   a.

   b.

   c.

4. A "medical patient" is a patient who is:
   a. hospitalized.
   c. critical.
   b. injured.
   d. ill.

5. A "trauma patient" is a patient who is:
   a. hospitalized.
   b. critical.
   c. injured.
   d. ill.

6. The "mechanism of injury" refers to the:
   a. patient's chief complaint.
   b. forces that caused an injury.
   c. mechanical advantage of the body.
   d. chronic condition the patient may have.

7. The "mechanism of injury" can NOT tell you:
   a. what injuries the patient may have.
   b. if the patient was ill before injury.
   c. how serious the patient's injuries may be.
   d. what patterns of injury you should suspect.

8. Kinetic energy is the total amount of energy:
   a. stored in an object at rest.
   b. in the velocity of an object.
   c. contained by an object in motion.
   d. contained in the mass of an object.

9. The more kinetic energy an object contains, the greater the damage it can cause when it impacts the body.

   _____ True

   _____ False

10. The higher the speed of an object, the more kinetic energy it has.

    _____ True

    _____ False

11. The amount of kinetic energy that is absorbed on impact depends on how much has been absorbed by other things first.

    _____ True

    _____ False

12. A person who falls on freshly plowed soil will be injured as severely as the person who falls the same distance onto cement pavement.

    _____ True

    _____ False

13. There are three basic types of impacts that occur when a car crashes into a tree. They are:

    a.

    b.

    c.

14. Down-and-under and up-and-over pathways of motion are associated with _____ collisions.
   a. head-on
   b. rollover
   c. rear-impact
   d. side-impact

15. Compare the patterns of injuries associated with the pathways of motion listed below.

Up-and-over:

Down-and-under:

16. Two cars involved in a head-on collision were traveling about 40 mph. The driver of a late-model sedan was wearing a lap and shoulder belt, and the car's air bag deployed on impact. His headrest was up. The driver of an old pickup truck was wearing only a lap belt. The seats of the truck have no headrests. As you approach the vehicles, you note major front-end damage to both. List the injuries you suspect each driver may suffer.

Driver of the sedan:

Driver of the pickup:

17. You arrive at the scene of a two-car collision. What injuries should you suspect in the driver whose car was broadsided?
    a. head and neck injuries
    b. chest injuries
    c. injury to the pelvis
    d. injury to the femur

18. A car is rear-ended by another vehicle and the driver of the car does not have his or her headrest up. Immediately suspect injury to the:
    a. clavicles.
    b. both carpals.
    c. cervical spine.
    d. tibia and fibula.

19. You find your patient unresponsive a few feet from his motorcycle. One side of the bike has large gashes in it, and the handlebar on that side has been snapped off. You find severe scrapes and cuts all along the patient's left side, and he has a swollen, deformed left lower leg. You suspect the mechanism of injury to be:
    a. ejection.
    b. head-on impact.
    c. angular impact.
    d. laying the bike down.

20. You respond to a six-year-old who has fallen 10 feet out of a tree. Her fall was broken by several branches. Which of the following would NOT help you to determine the severity of her injuries?
    a. distance of the fall
    b. body part that impacted first
    c. weight and height of the patient
    d. anything that interrupted the fall
    e. surface on which the patient landed

21. You are responding to the victim of a fall. You arrive on scene to learn that the patient fell 14 feet onto hard-packed dirt, landing face-down with initial contact to his abdomen and chest. Would you consider this a severe mechanism of injury? Why or why not?

22. Your patient has been stabbed. You should suspect a low-velocity injury that is at a site far from impact.

_____ True

_____ False

23. Your patient has been shot by a bullet from a handgun. You should suspect a high-velocity injury that affects tissues at the impact site only.

_____ True

_____ False

24. During the first, or primary, phase of an explosion, _____ typically causes injury.
    a. the fall onto a hard surface
    b. penetrating projectiles
    c. the pressure wave
    d. flying debris

25. Use the following clues to fill in the blanks. Then write the circled letters on the lines provided for "Unscrambled Letters." Unscramble the letters to find out what safety device is important for you and the general public.

    a. A headrest will prevent the head from whipping backward after this type of impact.

    ___ ___ (___) ___

    b. An impact to the top of the head can cause this type of fracture to the cervical spine.

    ___ ___ ___ ___ ___ (___) ___ ___ ___ ___ ___

    c. This minimizes injuries to a young child involved in a car accident.

    ___ ___ ___ (___) ___ ___ ___

    d. Seat belts and air bags help to protect motorists from serious injury in this type of collision.

    ___ (___) ___ ___ - ___ ___

    e. This abrupt stop to forward motion, such as occurs in a fall, can lead to serious injuries.

    ___ ___ ___ ___ (___) ___ ___ ___ ___ ___ ___ ___

    f. During a rollover, this may happen to an occupant who is not wearing a seat belt.

    ___ ___ ___ ___ (___) ___ ___ ___

    g. This is often called a "broadside" or "T-bone" collision.

    (___) ___ ___ ___ ___ ___ ___ ___ ___ ___

    h. This can be broken when the chest strikes the steering wheel.

    ___ (___) ___ ___ ___ ___ ___

    i. This event often results in three distinct phases, each with a typical pattern of injury.

    (___) ___ ___ ___ ___

Scrambled Letters: ____ ____ ____ ____ ____ ____ ____ ____ ____

Unscrambled Letters: ____ ____ ____ ____ ____ ____ ____ ____

CASE STUDY:
MOTOR-VEHICLE CRASH
▼

Read the following scenario and answer the questions that follow. Focus on the way in which the mechanisms of injury fit into the total picture.

You are responding to a vehicle collision in your rescue unit. When you arrive on scene you can see that four cars are involved. As you begin to unload equipment, a police officer tells you the story. A small pickup truck broke down in the middle of the roadway just over a rise. A station wagon coming over the rise at high speed rear-ended the truck. A pile-up ensued when a large sedan came upon the crash, locked its brakes, went into a sideways skid, and rolled three times. The sedan ended up over an embankment, the driver ejected. A fourth car, a foreign compact, managed to avoid the crash but slid sideways into a concrete barrier, striking the driver's side with no intrusion into the passenger space. Each car had one occupant. Each driver had taken safety precautions as follows:

- Pickup-truck driver wore a lap and shoulder belt, his headrest was up, and he had an air bag.
- Station-wagon driver wore a lap belt only and her headrest was up.
- Sedan driver had on no restraints of any kind and his headrest was down.
- Compact-car driver wore a lap and shoulder belt, her headrest was up, and she had an air bag.

26. You expect the driver of the station wagon to have taken either one of two pathways of motion. What are they?

27. Would the air bag have helped the driver of the compact car to avoid injury? Explain your answer.

28. Based on the mechanism of injury for each driver and the safety precautions each has taken, rank the four patients from most to least injured.

   a.

   b.

   c.

   d.

29. What injuries should you suspect in each of the drivers in the case study? Match the following injury patterns to the drivers.

   a. Suspect injuries to the left shoulder, left rib cage, and pelvis in the driver of the

   b. Suspect minor neck strain and a possible broken left clavicle in the driver of the

   c. Suspect lethal head and chest injuries in the driver of the

   d. Suspect major facial injuries, a broken sternum, and broken ribs in the driver of the

CHAPTER 10

PATIENT ASSESSMENT

KEY IDEAS

This chapter focuses on gathering accurate information about the patient's condition in order to provide the appropriate care. Key ideas include the following:

- First Responders must assess a patient's condition quickly and accurately using a step-by-step routine. This patient assessment routine will help you to focus on important concerns and establish patient care priorities. It also will help you to maintain self-control in stressful situations.

- The First Responder's patient assessment plan consists of a scene size-up, initial assessment, physical exam, patient history, ongoing assessment, and patient hand-off.

- There may be instances when you are unable to complete every aspect of the patient assessment plan because of priorities, such as establishing an airway or ventilating the patient. There will also be instances where you will be able to combine steps (for example, noting a patient's level of responsiveness as you assess his or her pulse).

- Whenever possible, use mnemonics such as "AVPU" (levels of responsiveness), "DOTS" (what to look for during a physical exam), and "SAMPLE" (information in the patient history) to help you remember important assessment steps.

- Noting changes in key areas—such as level of responsiveness and vital signs—can provide valuable information about your patient to other responders and the emergency room staff.

- A proper patient assessment and history will help you to make sense of the patient's condition and provide quality patient care.

1. What are the six steps of the First Responder's patient assessment plan?

   a.

   b.

   c.

   d.

   e.

   f.

2. The initial assessment is the most important part of the patient assessment plan because it identifies:
   a. life-threatening problems.
   b. the patient's medical history.
   c. potential long-term disabilities.
   d. painful, swollen, or deformed limbs.

3. Put a check next to the items that are included in the initial assessment:

   _____ a. examining the pupils

   _____ b. measuring blood pressure

   _____ c. assessing the patient's ABCs

   _____ d. forming a general impression

   _____ e. conducting a head-to-toe exam

   _____ f. assessing level of responsiveness

   _____ g. updating incoming EMS units

   _____ h. the patient's chief complaint

   _____ i. taking spinal precautions

4. You are responding to a 10-year-old patient who was struck by a car traveling 30 mph. The patient was thrown 25 feet onto the roadway. Number the following steps 1–7 to show the order in which they should be performed.

_____ Open and assess the airway.

_____ Check for serious external bleeding.

_____ Update EMS, and ask for the ETA of incoming units.

_____ Assess for approximate rate and rhythm of pulse.

_____ Manually stabilize the patient's head and neck.

_____ Introduce yourself and ask: "What happened? Where do you hurt?"
Tell the patient you are here to help.

_____ Assess for adequate rise and fall of the chest, ease of breathing, and adequate breathing rate.

5. You are managing a 62-year-old woman who collapsed at her office. Her airway is clear, and her respirations are 4–6 per minute and shallow. Her carotid pulse is slow and weak. Which of the following actions should you take?
   a. Do nothing, because the patient's ABCs are fine.
   b. Reassess the patient every three to five minutes.
   c. Respirations are too slow. Begin artificial ventilation.
   d. Begin CPR in order to support this patient's breathing.

6. The patient's _____ is the response to the question, "Can you tell me why you called EMS today?"
   a. chief complaint
   b. mechanism of injury
   c. level of responsiveness
   d. airway and breathing status

7. The AVPU mnemonic is helpful in describing a patient's level of responsiveness. Write the description beside each letter.

   A:

   V:

   P:

   U:

8. You are assessing a patient's mental status. The patient answers all your questions but does not offer any elaboration of his own. He appears to be distracted and in distress. Using the AVPU scale, how would you describe his level of responsiveness?
   a. alert
   b. verbal
   c. painful
   d. unresponsive

9. Several ice skaters collided, fell, and your patient was the guy on the bottom. He is responsive and, in fact, appears to be quite normal until you ask him, "What happened?" His response: "What do you mean?" Upon further questioning, you discover he does not recall the incident. Using the AVPU scale, what is this patient's level of responsiveness?
   a. alert
   b. verbal
   c. painful
   d. unresponsive

10. How would you assess the level of responsiveness in an adult whose mental status is normally altered?

11. How could you determine a 2-year-old's level of responsiveness?

12. You are managing a critically injured patient who has copious amounts of blood and broken teeth blocking her airway. You should:
    a. assess the airway and then move on to assess circulation.
    b. continue to try to clear the airway until you succeed.
    c. use forceful ventilations to try to clear the airway.
    d. reassess the airway every five minutes.

13. List three signs of adequate breathing:

    a.

    b.

    c.

14. To determine inadequate breathing look for all of the following EXCEPT:
    a. cyanosis.
    b. hemorrhaging.
    c. minimal chest rise.
    d. mental status changes.
    e. little or no air exhaled.
    f. extremely slow respirations.

15. If you determine that your patient's breathing is inadequate, you should:
    a. perform a head-to-toe exam.
    b. begin ventilating immediately.
    c. place him in a recovery position.
    d. ask bystanders if the patient was injured.

16. Generally, if your patient is a verbally responsive adult, use the _____ pulse to assess circulation.
   a. radial
   b. femoral
   c. carotid
   d. brachial

17. During the initial assessment of an unresponsive adult, use the _____ pulse to assess circulation.
   a. radial
   b. femoral
   c. carotid
   d. brachial

18. During the initial assessment, the pulse check for all infants is done at the _____ artery.
   a. radial
   b. femoral
   c. carotid
   d. brachial

19. If you find serious bleeding in your patient during the initial assessment, you should:
   a. phone or radio for help.
   b. control the blood flow immediately.
   c. provide CPR for one minute and then update EMS.
   d. reassess level of responsiveness and airway.

20. After the initial assessment of your patient, what information should you include in your update to EMS?

21. Write the numbers 1–6 to show the order in which you should perform the head-to-toe exam on an adult.

   _____ extremities

   _____ chest

   _____ head

   _____ pelvis

   _____ abdomen

   _____ neck

22. Read each scenario below. Then mark either "yes" or "no" to indicate whether or not you should perform a complete head-to-toe exam on the patient.

_____ a. Your patient has fallen 15 feet onto a concrete sidewalk.

_____ b. A 36-year-old man has accidentally cut his lower arm with a broken piece of glass.

_____ c. Your unresponsive patient has been found lying on a bench in the park.

23. There are three methods you should use to perform a physical exam. They are:

a.

b.

c.

24. The DOTS mnemonic can help you remember the signs of injury you are looking for during a physical exam. Write what each letter stands for.

D:

O:

T:

S:

25. For which of the following findings should you stop a head-to-toe exam to administer immediate care?
a. neck pain
b. tenderness to the groin
c. fracture to the lower arm
d. open wound to the leg with minimal bleeding

26. If you were to find an open wound of the chest in your patient, you should _____ immediately.
a. manually stabilize her head and neck
b. apply an occlusive (airtight) dressing
c. observe for deformities and tenderness
d. palpate the area around it for swelling

27. To assess circulation in the lower extremities, you should palpate the _____ and _____ pulse points.
a. dorsalis pedis, posterior tibial
b. brachial, dorsalis tibial
c. femoral, posterior pedis
d. brachial, femoral

28. Vital signs include the patient's:

a.

b.

c.

d.

e.

29. More important than any one vital sign is change in vital signs over time.

_____ True

_____ False

30. A respiration consists of _____ inhalation(s) and _____ exhalation(s).
   a. one-half, one-half
   b. only an, not an
   c. one, one
   d. two, two

31. A normal adult respiratory rate is _____ breaths per minute.
   a. 8–16
   b. 12–20
   c. 14–26
   d. 15–30
   e. 25–50

32. A normal respiratory rate for a child is _____ breaths per minute.
   a. 8–16
   b. 12–20
   c. 14–26
   d. 15–30
   e. 25–50

33. A normal respiratory rate for an infant is _____ breaths per minute.
   a. 8–16
   b. 12–20
   c. 14–26
   d. 15–30
   e. 25–50

34. To assess breathing properly, you should count the patient's respirations for _____ seconds and then multiply by _____ to get the respiratory rate.
   a. 40, 1
   b. 30, 2
   c. 15, 3
   d. 10, 4

35. A normal pulse rate for an adult is _____ per minute.
   a. 12–20
   b. 60–80
   c. 80–150
   d. 120–150

36. A normal pulse rate for a child is _____ per minute.
   a. 12-20
   b. 60-80
   c. 80-150
   d. 120-150

37. A normal pulse rate for an infant is _____ per minute.
   a. 12-20
   b. 60-80
   c. 80-150
   d. 120-150

38. If a patient's pulse rate is irregular or slow, count the beats for _____ seconds and then multiply by _____ to get an accurate reading.
   a. 40, 1
   b. 30, 2
   c. 15, 3
   d. 10, 4

39. Write what the following skin signs tell you about a patient's condition.

   a. Cool skin:

   b. Hot skin:

   c. Pale skin:

   d. Blueness:

   e. Black-and-blue mottling:

40. A reading of a patient's blood pressure can tell you:
   a. if pressure is being exerted by circulation.
   b. if the patient is an adult, child, or infant.
   c. how well pressure is being exerted in the body.
   d. how well the organs and tissues are being oxygenated.

41. Use the SAMPLE mnemonic to help you to remember important areas of questioning. Write what each letter stands for.

S:

A:

M:

P:

L:

E:

42. You are with an 81-year-old patient who is complaining of nausea, aching in all joints, weakness, and occasional dizziness. Are the patient's complaints signs or symptoms? Explain your answer.

43. You are with a 29-year-old medical patient who says he is "not feeling very well." Write two questions you might ask for the "S" part of a SAMPLE history.

44. You are waiting for the EMTs to arrive for an adult who is having trouble breathing. After you perform an initial assessment, the patient's problem appears to have eased considerably. You now are gathering a patient history. Write two questions you might ask for the "A" part of a SAMPLE history.

45. Your patient is elderly, confused, and frightened. A shop owner found her wandering in his store. She knows who she is and where she lives, but she cannot remember why she is in the store. After your initial assessment, you question her. What might you ask for the "M" part of a SAMPLE history?

46. You are with a 50-year-old patient who is having chest pain. What might you ask for the "P" part of a SAMPLE history?

47. Repeat the ongoing assessment every _____ minutes for an unstable patient and every _____ minutes for a stable one.
   a. 1, 10
   b. 5, 15
   c. 10, 20
   d. 15, 25

48. List the major elements of the patient hand-off report.

49. Joanne's patient hand-off report includes the following: "The patient's name is Pat O'Brien. He is 32 years old, and he has a painful and swollen right leg. Pat is alert with normal airway, breathing, and circulation. I've kept his leg manually stabilized in the position in which it was found for the last 10 minutes. Pat says his pain has been somewhat relieved." What information did Joanne omit from her report?

CASE STUDY: A CAR CRASH

▼

Read this scenario and answer the questions that follow. Focus specifically on the priorities of each of the major areas of patient assessment, from scene size-up through the patient hand-off report. Keep in mind that patient assessments answer the questions "What's going on with my patient? How can I help?" Continually ask yourself if the information you are gathering will help with the care of your patient's problem.

You are pulling a volunteer shift at the local firehouse late one night when you and one other First Responder are dispatched to a vehicle collision. You respond in the rescue truck and soon arrive at the scene of a single car rollover on a two-lane country road. There are no bystanders on scene. Your patient, a male in his forties, has been ejected from the car and lies in the roadway face up. As your partner quickly sets out flares to protect the scene, you confirm that there are no immediate scene dangers. Then you grab your jump kit and move to the patient's side. Your partner joins you and immediately stabilizes the patient's head and neck.

50. Your first task is to:
    a. assess airway, breathing, and circulation.
    b. inspect and palpate for any major injuries.
    c. determine if the patient has a chief complaint.
    d. find out from your dispatch the ETA of the ambulance.

51. As you kneel down beside the patient you note that he has snoring respirations and his tongue seems to be blocking his airway. The correct way to open his airway is to:
    a. perform a head-tilt/chin-lift maneuver.
    b. perform a jaw-thrust maneuver.
    c. use the recovery position so blood and vomit can drain more easily.
    d. hold his head in a neutral, in-line position.

As you continue to assess the patient, you talk to him. He responds by calling out, speaking incoherently, and moaning. His breathing appears to be very labored and rapid. His pulse is thready, rapid, and very weak.

52. Based on this information, use the AVPU scale to describe the patient's level of responsiveness.

53. As you begin your head-to-toe exam, your patient, who had been moaning and shouting, now becomes very quiet. What should your first action be?

If you have time before the EMTs arrive, how will you perform a head-to-toe exam on this patient? Beside each area of the body, write what you would do.

54. Head:

     D:

     O:

     T:

     S:

55. Neck:

     D:

     O:

     T:

     S:

56. Chest:

     D:

     O:

     T:

     S:

57. Abdomen:

     D:

     O:

     T:

     S:

58. Back (posterior):

    D:

    O:

    T:

    S:

59. Pelvis:

    D:

    O:

    T:

    S:

60. Extremities:

    D:

    O:

    T:

    S:

CHAPTER 11

COMMUNICATION AND DOCUMENTATION

KEY IDEAS

This chapter provides additional information on the types of communication and documentation expected of a First Responder. Key ideas include the following:

- First Responders have opportunities to communicate with other EMS personnel on the radio or phone as well as in person. These communications must be accurate, complete, brief, and to the point.

- First Responders must report to dispatch when en route to a call, upon arrival on scene, when additional assistance is needed, and when they return to service.

- Good communication skills can help First Responders get the information they need to provide—and help others to provide—proper emergency care to the patient.

- A prehospital care report is used to transfer patient information from one person to another, to provide legal documentation, and to improve the EMS system.

- Special incident reports may be required for infectious disease exposure, injury to EMS personnel, conflicts between agencies, and multiple-casualty incidents.

CONTENT REVIEW

▼

1. Complete the sentence by circling the letters beside all of the correct answers.

   A First Responder is expected to:
   a. update incoming EMS units.
   b. request help from EMS dispatch.
   c. reassure and comfort the patient.
   d. ask medical direction for advice.
   e. provide a hand-off report to EMTs.
   f. obtain the patient's medical history.
   g. determine the patient's chief complaint.

2. Match the components of a radio system with the correct descriptions.

   Base station •   • Radio mounted in a vehicle

   Mobile radio •   • Rebroadcasts radio transmissions

   Portable radio •   • Hand-held radio

   Repeater •   • Stationary radio located in a dispatch center or hospital

3. You are in your unit and have just pulled out of the station to respond to a "man down" at a public park. You pick up your radio mike and report you are:
   a. on scene.
   b. en route to the scene.
   c. available for the next call.
   d. in need of additional assistance.

4. When using a radio microphone, you should talk with your mouth ____ from the mike.
   a. $\frac{1}{8}$ to $\frac{1}{4}$ inch
   b. two to three inches
   c. as far away as possible
   d. about an arm-length away

5. Write five "rules" you should follow while talking on your radio.

   a.

   b.

   c.

   d.

   e.

6. You observe a rescuer call for medical direction. He introduces himself by identifying his unit and the fact that he is a First Responder. He briefly outlines the reasons he is calling. Then he provides a brief pertinent history including the results of a physical exam, plus the treatment he provided and the patient's reaction to it. What did he leave out?

7. The effectiveness of communication with a patient can depend on your tone of voice, your body language, and your approach. Four possible approaches are defined below. Write the approach taken for each of the quotes that follow.

   "Teacher" — provide information and explain things.
   "Friend" — comfort, sympathize, be empathetic.
   "Authority" — take control, dictate how the call will progress.
   "Advisor" — give advice and persuade, convince the patient.

   _____ **a.** "From what I can tell, this swelling and deformity may indicate a broken bone."

   _____ **b.** "I'm so sorry that you are in pain. Is there anything I can do to ease it?"

   _____ **c.** "If you decide not to go to the hospital, it will be necessary to get the police department involved. It is imperative that you go to the hospital."

   _____ **d.** "I really think you ought to go to the hospital. Look at how much your family is worried. If they are worried enough to call 9-1-1, then it seems to me that you really ought to be checked out."

   _____ **e.** "Tell you what. Let's go to the hospital and get that cut stitched up, and then you will be in a better position to make a decision about what to do with your damaged car. Won't you feel better if we get your injuries taken care of first?"

   _____ **f.** "I can just bet that your neck hurts. I realize that lying on this backboard is no fun either. You will be at the hospital soon. Hopefully, a doctor can get you out of this contraption quickly."

   _____ **g.** "At this point, I haven't found any serious injuries on your child. His vital signs appear quite stable, too. The doctor at the emergency department may want to run some tests to make sure everything is okay."

   _____ **h.** "Here's the plan. The only way we can get you out of this car is if you hold still while the fire department uses a pry bar to get this door open. You need to hold still."

8. List three reasons why a prehospital care report is used by First Responders.

    a.

    b.

    c.

9. Your patient, Mr. O'Brien, is refusing further care even though you feel it is necessary for him. What should you document on your run report about this?

10. Identify the situations listed below that require special documentation.

    _____ **a.** exposure to blood or body fluids

    _____ **b.** interagency conflict

    _____ **c.** motorcycle collision

    _____ **d.** train derailment with 25 passengers

    _____ **e.** child who choked on a hotdog

CASE STUDY: THE PCR

Read the scenario that follows. Then fill out the prehospital care report provided. If necessary, use an additional sheet of paper for further narrative.

You are showing your new partner the ropes of East Lydius Fire and Rescue Squad when a call comes in for a single-car motor-vehicle collision at the intersection of First and Division Streets. A passerby reports that a guy drove his car right into a tree.

As you arrive at the scene, you can see that this is a residential street with very little traffic. Your partner says, "This is gonna be bad. The posted speed limit is 30 mph and there are no skid marks. Good thing there are no wires or tree limbs down."

When it is safe to approach, you see a young man of about 25, who is seated behind the wheel of the car. The car engine is off. You take the key out. The patient is wearing his seatbelt and the airbag is deployed. The front end of the car has some minor damage. The windshield is intact.

Several empty beer cans are on the back floor. You ask him if he is okay and his answer is garbled. Your partner manually stabilizes the patient's head and neck, while you talk with him and check him over. The patient continues to answer your questions, and his speech is becoming easier to understand. He says his name is Andy Kohn and that he has a terrible headache but that nothing else hurts him. Breathing is unlabored at 18 breaths per minute with good air movement and no odor of food or beverage on the breath. You apply oxygen via nonrebreather mask. His radial pulse is strong at a rate of 68.

The patient asks if anyone else is hurt and if his car will be okay. As you prepare to take his blood pressure, you see a Medic Alert bracelet that says your patient is medically followed by Dr. Cullen for a seizure disorder.

Your patient tells you that he is pretty fortunate as generally he is never sick, but that he ran out of his medicine for his convulsions and was on his way to the drug store for a refill. The patient's speech is now clear and his headache is nearly gone. The EMTs arrive and you give them a hand-off report and say "Goodbye. Good luck" to your patient.

First Responder Prehospital Care Report

REMO

M	D	Y

DATE

AGENCY CODE

RUN NO.

CALL REC'D

ENROUTE

AT SCENE

IN SERVICE

NAME

ADDRESS

NEXT OF KIN

PHYSICIAN

VEH. ID.

AGENCY NAME

DOB   SEX M F   Ph#

CALL LOCATION

CHIEF COMPLAINT

CALL TYPE

PAST MEDICAL HISTORY		TIME	RESP.	PULSE	B.P.	CONS
❏ HYPERTENSION ❏ STROKE ❏ SEIZURES ❏ DIABETES ❏ COPD ❏ CARDIAC ❏ ALLERGY ❏ OTHER ❏ MEDICATION (LIST IN COMMENTS)	V I T A L		RATE ❏ Regular ❏ Shallow ❏ Labored	❏ Regular ❏ Irregular		
	S I G N S		RATE ❏ Regular ❏ Shallow ❏ Labored	❏ Regular ❏ Irregular		

PHYSICAL EXAM FINDINGS

TREATMENT GIVEN

DISPOSITION (SEE LIST)

DISP. CODE

CREW

NAME   DRIVER   ❏ EMT ❏ AEMT #

NAME   ❏ EMT ❏ AEMT #

NAME   ❏ EMT ❏ AEMT #

© Regional Emergency Medical Organization, Albany, NY

CHAPTER 12

CARDIAC AND RESPIRATORY EMERGENCIES

KEY IDEAS

This chapter describes the signs, symptoms, and emergency care of cardiac and respiratory emergencies. Key ideas include the following:

- Any adult with pain or discomfort to the chest, neck, shoulder, arm, or jaw should be suspected of having a heart attack.

- Emergency care for patients with chest pain focuses on supporting the patient's ABCs, comforting the patient, and activating EMS as quickly as possible.

- Specific cardiac conditions include angina pectoris and acute myocardial infarction.

- Rapid treatment is necessary when disease or injury affects the body's ability to obtain oxygen.

- Respiratory distress occurs when air cannot pass easily into the lungs or has difficulty passing out of the lungs.

- Emergency care of a patient in respiratory distress focuses on supporting the patient's airway and breathing, helping the patient find a position of comfort, and activating EMS as quickly as possible.

- Specific causes of respiratory emergencies include chronic obstructive pulmonary disease, asthma, pneumonia, acute pulmonary edema, and hyperventilation.

1. Coronary artery disease:
   a. narrows the coronary artery.
   b. is unrelated to arteriosclerosis.
   c. reduces bodily pain and discomfort.
   d. increases the oxygen that goes to the heart.

2. List eight risk factors for coronary artery disease.

   a.

   b.

   c.

   d.

   e.

   f.

   g.

   h.

3. List five signs and symptoms that may indicate a patient has a cardiac problem.

   a.

   b.

   c.

   d.

   e.

4. Using the mnemonic OPQRRRST can help you to:
   a. get a good description of the patient's pain.
   b. perform a thorough head-to-toe physical exam.
   c. obtain a complete and relevant patient history.
   d. examine the patient for life-threatening conditions.

5. Write the word that each letter in the mnemonic helps you to recall.

O:

P:

Q:

R:

R:

R:

S:

T:

6. When you are managing a patient with a possible cardiac emergency, you should activate the EMS system:
   a. after completing a head-to-toe exam.
   b. as soon as chest pain is recognized.
   c. after gathering an accurate patient history.
   d. if the patient truly is having a heart attack.

7. You find your neighbor sitting on a couch, stating that he's having chest pain and difficulty breathing. After you activate the EMS system, you begin to comfort and reassure the patient. You then perform the following steps. Number them 1–6 in the correct order.

_____ **a.** Gather a patient history.

_____ **b.** Perform an initial assessment.

_____ **c.** Place him in a position of comfort.

_____ **d.** Have the patient cease all movement.

_____ **e.** Administer high-flow oxygen by way of a nonrebreather mask.

_____ **f.** Monitor the patient carefully, and be prepared to perform CPR if necessary.

8. The emergency care of angina and myocardial infarction is the same as for any patient with chest pain.

_____ True

_____ False

9. Check all the items below that are true about angina:

_____ **a.** It can appear suddenly.

_____ **b.** Stress can be the cause of it.

_____ **c.** Sometimes it has no apparent cause.

_____ **d.** It causes permanent damage to the heart.

_____ **e.** Usually it is associated with physical exertion.

_____ **f.** You can tell the difference between it and a heart attack.

_____ **g.** If left untreated, it could cause a heart attack.

10. Identify all the statements that are true about myocardial infarction.
    a. It means permanent death of heart muscle.
    b. It is easily distinguishable from angina.
    c. It can occur when blood to the heart is greatly reduced.
    d. It commonly occurs as a result of coronary artery disease.

11. Identify all the symptoms of chest discomfort associated with a cardiac emergency.
    a. heaviness or squeezing in the chest
    b. mild to severe crushing pain
    c. numbness in the chest
    d. acute indigestion

12. The most common symptom of heart attack is respiratory distress.

_____ True

_____ False

13. You respond in your rescue unit to an "unknown medical problem." You find a 63-year-old woman who says that she is experiencing nausea, dizziness, and slight shortness of breath. These symptoms came on suddenly while she was watching television. She has a history of "heart problems" and edema in her legs but has never had a heart attack. She says she recently got over the flu. Your partner turns to you and says, "Sounds like the flu to me. She's not having any chest pain, so I don't think she's having a cardiac problem." Agree? Disagree? Explain.

14. List seven general signs and symptoms of respiratory distress.

    a.

    b.

    c.

    d.

    e.

    f.

    g.

15. List five general guidelines for emergency care of a patient in respiratory distress.

    a.

    b.

    c.

    d.

    e.

16. A patient in the "tripod" position may be described as someone who is sitting _____ and fighting to breathe.
    a. bolt upright, leaning forward
    b. bent over, head between knees
    c. with one leg forward, one leg back
    d. splinting the chest with both arms

17. You and your partner respond to a 67-year-old male complaining of shortness of breath. He suffers from emphysema. You find your patient sitting bolt upright, speaking in two- and three-word sentences, breathing 36 times per minute, so you apply high-flow oxygen by nonrebreather mask. Your partner states: "Remember, this guy may be a hypoxic-drive breather. We need to keep his oxygen at four liters per minute by cannula. We don't want him to stop breathing." Agree? Disagree? Explain.

18. Identify all the conditions listed below that can cause wheezing.
    a. asthma
    b. chronic bronchitis
    c. smoke inhalation
    d. acute congestive heart failure
    e. severe allergic reaction
    f. acute pulmonary embolism

19. Which two of the following quotes about hyperventilation are accurate?
    a. "Oxygen should never be applied to these patients. It can make them worse."
    b. "Not everyone who is breathing rapidly or deeply is hyperventilating."
    c. "When patients hyperventilate, they exhale too much carbon dioxide."
    d. "Putting a paper bag over a hyperventilator's face will cure most cases of hyperventilation."

CASE STUDY: PATIENT WITH A CARDIAC EMERGENCY

Read the scenario and answer the questions that follow. Remember that heart attacks and other cardiac emergencies can present with a variety of signs and symptoms.

After activating the EMS system, you respond to the eighth hole of the local golf course where a male in his 60s has reportedly collapsed. You arrive at the green and are pulling your jump kit out of the back of the golf cart when one of the patient's friends approaches you. "I kept telling George that he ought to get out of the sun and take a break, but he wouldn't listen. He's got a heart problem. They put a pacemaker in a couple of years ago. We were just finishing this hole when he sort of grabbed his chest, stumbled, and passed out on the green."

You approach the patient, who is lying on his side on the green, concerned friends around him. "Is George awake?" you ask.

"I don't think so," answers one of his friends.

20. Your first action should be to:
    a. open George's airway.
    b. check George for a pulse.
    c. confirm that George is still breathing.
    d. determine George's level of responsiveness.

You find that George is awake but very anxious, with a patent airway, respirations 32, pulse 32, and blood pressure 66/32. His skin is pale, cool, and moist.

21. George should probably be placed in which of the following positions?
    a. shock position
    b. prone position
    c. recovery position
    d. position of comfort

22. You attempt to place a nonrebreather mask on George. He is quite combative and tries to prevent you from placing the mask on his face. Why is George so combative?

23. After you have applied oxygen, you attempt to gather a patient history. List at least five questions to which you should get answers.

a.

b.

c.

d.

e.

24. As you are gathering a patient history from the patient, he suddenly becomes very quiet. "George?" you call to him. There is no answer. "George!" you shout. Still there is no answer. To decide if you have to perform CPR, you must perform the following steps. Number them 1–7 in the correct order.

_____ **a.** Lay George flat on his back on the golf green.

_____ **b.** Give two slow, full breaths.

_____ **c.** Check the carotid pulse and determine pulselessness.

_____ **d.** Open the airway.

_____ **e.** Begin CPR.

_____ **f.** Determine that George is not breathing.

_____ **g.** Shake George to verify unresponsiveness.

25. As you start CPR, you notice that you are not getting any chest rise with ventilations. What should your first action be?

26. You have an automatic external defibrillator with you. At what point should you attempt to patch George into the machine? Explain your decision.

27. You manage to turn CPR over to a bystander and are able to set up the defibrillator. As directed, you deliver three shocks to George's heart. You are able to feel a carotid pulse, so you continue with artificial ventilation until the paramedics arrive. After they take over, you give them a report. Write your hand-off report below, being sure to include your original assessment of George, his status change, and the care you provided.

CHAPTER 13

OTHER COMMON MEDICAL COMPLAINTS

KEY IDEAS
▼

This chapter focuses on common medical complaints other than cardiac and respiratory emergencies. These complaints include altered mental status, hyperglycemia and hypoglycemia, poisoning, stroke, seizures, and abdominal pain and distress. Key ideas include the following:

- Altered mental status can range from mildly disoriented to combative to unresponsive. An accurate history should include when the patient last ate, what type of medication the patient has taken, and when it was taken. This information can give the hospital staff clues to the underlying problem. First Responder care focuses on assessing and monitoring the patient's airway and breathing, and administering oxygen if you are allowed.

- Treatment for both hyperglycemia and hypoglycemia focuses on supporting the patient's airway and breathing and, if your EMS system allows, the administration of sugar.

- An accurate history of a poisoning includes determining the route of the poisoning, the amount of poison that has entered the patient's body, and when the exposure occurred. Your top priority in a poisoning emergency is the patient's airway. If EMS resources are delayed, call your regional poison control center or medical direction for instructions.

- Signs and symptoms of stroke range from altered mental status to loss of motor function and unresponsiveness. Treatment for stroke focuses on maintaining the patient's airway and breathing.

- Seizures may last five minutes or they may be prolonged. They are rarely life-threatening, but they do indicate a very serious condition. Treatment for seizures focuses on maintaining the patient's airway and breathing, and protecting the patient from injury.

- All abdominal pain should be taken seriously. Any abdominal pain that is persistent or is significant enough for the patient or family to call for assistance should be considered an emergency. Treatment consists of assuring the patient's airway and breathings, administering oxygen if possible, and staying alert for signs of shock.

▼

1. When your patient's chief complaint is as general as "I feel weak," you should proceed with your patient assessment plan and emergency care the same as you would for any patient.

    _____ True

    _____ False

2. Describe emergency care for a patient who has a general complaint such as "I don't feel well."

3. When a patient finds it difficult to understand what you are saying, he has an altered mental status.

    _____ True

    _____ False

4. Sometimes unusual responses or unusual behaviors are normal for a patient.

    _____ True

    _____ False

5. Identify from the list below all the possible causes of altered mental status.
    a. Decreased levels of oxygen in the blood
    b. Low blood sugar
    c. Stroke
    d. Seizures
    e. Fever
    f. Infection
    g. Poisoning
    h. Head injury
    i. Psychiatric conditions

6. What questions might you ask to find out if your patient has an altered mental status?

7. Check all the items below that are true about your care of patients with altered mental status.

_____ **a.** Don't frighten them by saying you called an ambulance.

_____ **b.** Avoid asking questions to get a patient history.

_____ **c.** Be gentle and empathetic, truthful and kind.

_____ **d.** Explain that everything will be all right.

8. It's about 2:00 in the afternoon. You and your partner spot two young men in their 20s standing in front of a bar. One of them waves you over. "Hey, this is my friend Matt. He isn't acting right. He looks drunk, but I've been with him all night and we only had a couple of beers." When you ask the patient what's wrong, he tells you he's feeling dizzy. You observe that his speech is slurred and he is staggering. How should you proceed?

9. Why is it especially important to get an accurate history from a patient with an altered mental status?

10. The human body needs both oxygen and sugar to produce the energy that sustains it.

_____ True

_____ False

11. You and your partner are managing a patient with an altered mental status. The patient has a history of diabetes. You move to apply oxygen to the patient, and your partner says, "Don't bother. This guy is a diabetic. He needs sugar, not oxygen." Do you agree or disagree with this statement? Explain your answer.

12. A condition in which a patient has too much insulin or too little blood sugar is called:
  a. hypothermia.
  b. hypoglycemia.
  c. hyperglycemia.
  d. hyperchondria.

13. A condition in which a patient has too little insulin and too much blood sugar is called:
  a. hypothermia.
  b. hypoglycemia.
  c. hyperglycemia.
  d. hyperchondria.

14. When blood sugar is too low or too high, the body reacts. The most common reaction is:

15. Decide whether each patient described may be suffering from hypoglycemia or hyperglycemia. Write in the spaces provided.

_____ **a.** A patient takes more than the prescribed dose of insulin.

_____ **b.** A patient exercises more strenuously than usual.

_____ **c.** A patient with diabetes injects too little insulin.

_____ **d.** A patient eats too many sugary foods.

_____ **e.** A patient skips lunch in preparation for a big dinner.

_____ **f.** A patient suffers a viral respiratory infection.

16. Write nine signs and symptoms that could indicate a patient is suffering from hypoglycemia or hyperglycemia.

a.

b.

c.

d.

e.

f.

g.

h.

i.

17. During scene size-up, what four observations might you make in the home of a patient who has diabetes?

a.

b.

c.

d.

18. You are assessing a 28-year-old man who is wearing a medallion around his neck which says he has diabetes. He was found wandering aimlessly in the street. He is now awake but slightly confused and slow to answer your questions. List five questions you could ask this patient to gather information about his emergency.

a.

b.

c.

d.

e.

19. Describe the rule regarding administering sugar to patients. Is it necessary to confirm that the patient is specifically hypoglycemic or hyperglycemic before administering sugar? Explain.

20. List four major routes by which patients are poisoned, and give an example for each.

a.

b.

c.

d.

21. Your neighbor has just banged on your door, stating that her two-year-old ate a handful of mouse poison. You call 9-1-1 and run over to your neighbor's house to help. List four questions you would ask your neighbor in order to gather a good patient history about the event.

a.

b.

c.

d.

22. In which one or more of the following patients should you NOT induce vomiting?
   a. one who is unresponsive
   b. one who has swallowed a petroleum-based solvent
   c. one who cannot maintain his or her own airway
   d. one who is pregnant

23. Activated charcoal may be used with syrup of ipecac in cases of severe poisoning.

_____ True

_____ False

24. Activated charcoal:
   a. is effective against all inhaled and injected poisons.
   b. is very absorbent and binds with poisons in the stomach.
   c. may be effective five hours after poison ingestion.
   d. should be given along with syrup of ipecac.

25. Common signs and symptoms of poisoning by absorption include all of the following EXCEPT:
    a. itching or irritation.
    b. redness, rash, or blisters.
    c. abdominal pain or discomfort.
    d. liquid or powder on the skin.

26. Rescuers have responded to an attempted suicide. They are told that the patient has closed up her garage and is sitting in her car with the engine idling. What should be the rescuers' first action?
    a. Remove the patient from the garage immediately.
    b. Attempt to ventilate the garage.
    c. Don a self-contained breathing apparatus.
    d. Apply 100% oxygen to the patient.

27. You have responded to a residence where it appears that a woman in her 40s has been exposed to carbon monoxide from a faulty kerosene heater. She is experiencing headaches, dizziness, and chest tightness. Since she has been removed from the house, she states that her symptoms are clearing up. Your partner says that he feels okay releasing her to follow up with her personal physician. Do you agree or disagree with this decision? Explain.

28. Patients who are at risk for stroke include:

    a.

    b.

    c.

29. Explain the difference between a transient ischemic attack (TIA) and a stroke.

30. List three types of signs or symptoms a patient who has had a stroke might exhibit. Give an example of each one.

a.

b.

c.

31. Evaluate the following statements regarding stroke and the treatment for stroke. Write "agree" or "disagree" beneath each one. If you disagree with the statement, explain.

a. Provide the same emergency care you would provide to any patient with an altered mental status.

b. You need not be especially alert to the patient's airway or breathing status, because stroke usually affects only the limbs, speech, or facial muscles.

c. If you suspect stroke in a patient, take a carotid pulse and radial pulse on both sides of the body.

d. Do not talk to the stroke patient during emergency care, especially if the patient cannot communicate. His or her inability to respond to you will only frighten the patient further.

32. Read the statements below. Which ones are NOT appropriate to make in front of a stroke patient?
    a. It looks like this patient had "the big one." Weird vital signs, paralysis on one side. . . Nope, Mr. Gonzalez does not look good.
    b. Mr. Gonzalez, I can see that you are having trouble speaking. I'll be able to provide you with better care if you try harder to speak more clearly.
    c. Mr. Gonzalez, I think you are having a stroke. It looks like it's pretty bad, so I'm going to take you to the hospital.
    d. Mr. Gonzalez, let's take a ride over to the hospital. I know that you're concerned about not being able to speak clearly, so I'm going to have a doctor check you out.

33. Of all causes of seizure, which one is the most common in infants and children?
    a. hypoglycemia
    b. stroke
    c. infection
    d. fever

34. Identify two items that are true of status epilepticus:
    a. two or three seizures occurring within a few hours of one another
    b. a single seizure lasting longer than 30 minutes
    c. a series of seizures in rapid progression with no period of responsiveness between them
    d. a single seizure lasting longer than 10 minutes

35. The post-seizure phase is characterized by:
    a. unusual smell or flash of light that lasts a split second.
    b. unresponsiveness followed by extreme muscle rigidity.
    c. violent jerking of the arms and legs.
    d. deep sleep with gradual recovery.

36. You have responded to a six-year-old with possible seizures. One of the parents tells you that the child has been having seizures "on and off for most of the day." When you inquire about what the seizures look like, he tells you: "Oh, he's probably had 10 to 20 seizures today." Your partner grows quite concerned, states, "Sounds like status epilepticus to me," and rushes off to get the airway and oxygen equipment. Does his response seem appropriate? Why or why not?

37. List at least four questions that will help you gather pertinent information about a seizure patient.

a.

b.

c.

d.

38. You have responded to a man reportedly in seizure. You arrive at the entrance to an alleyway and notice a patient lying against a building about 30 feet away, still in seizure. A witness tells you that the patient fell to the ground and struck his head when his seizure began. Number the following actions 1–6 to correctly order the steps for managing this patient.

_____ **a.** Perform a head-to-toe physical exam to look for any trauma, incontinence, medical alert bracelets, etc.

_____ **b.** Size up the scene. Check for hazards and any clues that might explain his seizures.

_____ **c.** Protect the patient's head until the seizure stops.

_____ **d.** When the seizure stops, provide manual stabilization of the patient's head and neck.

_____ **e.** Attempt to gather medical history from the patient.

_____ **f.** Perform an initial assessment and provide treatment as appropriate.

39. Describe the type of approach you think would be most effective for communicating with a post-seizure patient who is still somewhat disoriented.

40. List six signs and symptoms of abdominal pain and distress.

a.

b.

c.

d.

e.

f.

41. When you palpate your patient's abdomen, he turns away from you and draws his knees toward his chest. What is this called? What does it signify?

42. Check all the items listed below that refer to a proper assessment of a patient with abdominal distress.

_____ **a.** The initial assessment is the first priority.

_____ **b.** Gather a good patient history.

_____ **c.** Determine whether the patient is restless or quiet.

_____ **d.** Find out if movement causes pain.

_____ **e.** Check to see if the abdomen is distended.

_____ **f.** Note if the patient can relax the abdominal wall.

_____ **g.** Palpate the abdomen gently.

_____ **h.** Examine the area of pain first.

_____ **i.** Determine if the abdomen is rigid or soft.

_____ **j.** Stay alert for signs of shock.

43. Your patient is suffering from abdominal pain and is complaining of feeling nauseated. If appropriate, you should place the patient in a _____ position.
   a. supine
   b. left lateral
   c. prone
   d. shock

CASE STUDY: TIA OR CVA

Read the following case study and answer the questions that follow. Pay attention to the signs and symptoms that indicate this patient has experienced some type of significant brain problem.

It's dinnertime at the station. You and the rest of the volunteer fire squad are getting ready to sit down to finish off a kettle full of spaghetti when you are dispatched to a "male in his 60s, unknown medical problem." You arrive at a residence and are flagged down by the patient's wife. "John just collapsed in the kitchen," she states as you pull your equipment from the truck. "He's awake now, but he doesn't seem right. Nothing like this has ever happened before."

She tells you that John was washing his hands at the sink when he stumbled back against a counter and slid down to a sitting position. He "just stared off into space" for at least a minute. He then appeared to become somewhat aware of his surroundings, but was unable to speak or move his left side. You find John still sitting on the kitchen floor. He looks at you as you approach, but does not speak.

44. After taking BSI precautions, you should assess John's:
   a. pupils and blood pressure.
   b. carotid or radial pulse.
   c. level of responsiveness.
   d. airway and breathing.

As you complete your assessment of John, you find he is able to move all extremities and he has begun to speak clearly. "What happened, Grace?" he asks his wife.

45. Describe a life-threatening condition that could occur to John based on what you know about his condition.

46. After a few minutes, you observe that John seems to be responding better. He seems to be alert and able to speak. List five questions that you could ask him in order to better understand his collapse and current condition.

a.

b.

c.

d.

e.

47. After establishing that John is alert and oriented, what other signs or symptoms should you reassess?

48. When the EMT-Paramedics arrive, they take over emergency care of John. He tells them that he feels fine and does not want to wear any oxygen or go to the hospital. Do you agree with him? Back up your answer with an explanation.

CHAPTER 14

HEAT AND COLD EMERGENCIES

KEY IDEAS

This chapter focuses on recognizing the causes, signs and symptoms, and emergency care of heat and cold emergencies. Key ideas include the following:

- The human body is constantly trying to maintain its average core temperature of around 98.6°F.

- In the cold, the body holds onto its heat by constricting blood vessels near its surface. Also, hair erects, thickening the layer of warm air trapped near the skin. The body can produce more heat, if needed, by shivering and by producing certain hormones such as epinephrine.

- The body loses heat through convection, conduction, radiation, evaporation, and respiration.

- Cold-related emergencies include generalized hypothermia and local cold injuries. Treatment focuses on supporting the patient's ABCs and rewarming as appropriate.

- Heat-related emergencies include heat cramps, heat exhaustion, and heat stroke. Treatment for these emergencies focuses on supporting the patient's ABCs and cooling the patient as necessary.

CONTENT REVIEW

▼

1. Match the following terms with their correct definitions and examples. Each term may be used more than once.

   convection   conduction   radiation   evaporation

   _____ a. This is the transfer of heat from the surface of one object to the surface of another object without physical contact.

   _____ b. Heat loss occurs through this process when one sweats.

   _____ c. Cold air that touches the skin is warmed and then replaced by other, cooler molecules of air.

   _____ d. Wind chill relates to this process.

   _____ e. Body heat is pulled away 240 times faster by this process when one's clothes are wet.

   _____ f. Covering the head, hands, and feet will reduce heat loss through this method.

   _____ g. This method of heat loss is only effective when air humidity is relatively low.

2. Shivering is:
   a. a normal finding in hyperthermia.
   b. the body's attempt to generate heat.
   c. a sign of the brain being deprived of oxygen.
   d. a life threat.

3. When the body loses more heat than it can produce, _____ may occur.
   a. hypoglycemia
   b. hyperthermia
   c. hypothermia
   d. hyperglycemia

4. There are five stages of hypothermia. Each one can progress to the next, more serious stage. Number the stages 1–5 to show the order of worsening hypothermia.

   _____ a. apathy and decreased muscle function

   _____ b. decreased level of responsiveness

   _____ c. death

   _____ d. decreased vital signs

   _____ e. shivering

5. Infants and children are better able to maintain body temperature than adults are.

_____ True

_____ False

6. When managing an unresponsive hypothermic patient, check the pulse for _____ seconds before starting CPR.
  a. 15
  b. 30
  c. 45
  d. 60

7. Your patient is a 35-year-old woman who was found stumbling along a hiker's trail. She is slightly disoriented and complaining of stiff joints and weakness. She appears to be clumsy, confused, and forgetful. Her skin is cold to the touch. Given this information, list five questions you would want to ask for a SAMPLE history.

  a.

  b.

  c.

  d.

  e.

8. Identify the three items that do NOT tell how to care for a patient with generalized hypothermia.
  a. Massage cold extremities gently.
  b. Comfort, calm, and reassure the patient.
  c. Have the patient sip a hot drink or hot soup.
  d. Remove the patient from the cold environment.
  e. Administer warm, humidified oxygen if possible.
  f. Allow the patient to walk to stimulate circulation.
  g. Remove wet clothing, and cover the patient with a blanket.

9. Exposure to extreme cold for a short time or moderate cold for a long time can cause hyperthermia.

_____ True

_____ False

10. List three risk factors that contribute to a patient's vulnerability to generalized hypothermia.

  a.

  b.

  c.

11. Complete the sentence: Because hypothermic patients with temperatures as low as 60°F have

been resuscitated, EMS personnel have been known to say, "You're not dead until you're

_____ and dead."

12. The patient with mild hypothermia will present with _____ and will still be alert.
   a. cold skin and shivering
   b. fixed and dilated pupils
   c. extremely slow pulse rate
   d. extremely slow breathing rate

13. It is recommended that heat packs be applied to the neck, armpits, and groin of a mildly hypothermic patient.

   _____ True

   _____ False

14. Indicate whether each sentence describes mild hypothermia or severe hypothermia. Write "mild" or "severe" beside each one.

   _____ a. Patient is shivering uncontrollably.

   _____ b. Patient states he is quite cold.

   _____ c. Patient is awake but disoriented as to person, place, and time.

   _____ d. Patient responds to questions slowly but appropriately.

   _____ e. Patient has a slowed pulse rate and respiratory rate.

   _____ f. Patient has an increased pulse rate and blood pressure.

   _____ g. Patient's speech does not make sense.

   _____ h. Patient's movements are normal but uncoordinated.

   _____ i. Patient has muscular rigidity.

15. You are extricating a severely hypothermic patient from a mountainous region. As you are lifting the stretcher into the ambulance, one member of the rescue party accidentally slams the side of the stretcher. Your partner shouts, "Hey! Be more careful! What are you trying to do, kill the guy?" Why would your partner say this? Why is it so important to handle a severely hypothermic patient gently?

16. A sign of an early or superficial local cold injury is:
    a. swelling and blistering.
    b. mottled and cyanotic skin.
    c. the skin is firm to the touch.
    d. blanching when skin is touched lightly.

17. Care of a late or deep local cold injury includes all of the following EXCEPT:
    a. rewarm it by soaking in 105°F water.
    b. cover it with a dry cloth or dressings.
    c. manually stabilize the injured extremity.
    d. monitor the patient for signs of hypothermia.

18. When the body cannot get rid of excess heat, _____ may occur.
    a. hypoglycemia
    b. hyperthermia
    c. hypothermia
    d. hyperglycemia

19. Explain briefly how each factor listed below contributes to hyperthermia.

    a. Climate:

    b. Exercise and activity:

    c. Drugs and alcohol:

    d. Age and medical condition:

20. List five signs and symptoms of a heat-related emergency.

    a.

    b.

    c.

    d.

    e.

21. A patient with moist, pale, and normal-to-cool skin has the very serious and life-threatening condition known as heat stroke.

_____ True

_____ False

22. You are managing a 27-year-old runner who has dropped out of a mini-marathon after becoming dizzy and nauseous. He presents with pale, cool, and extremely wet skin, headache, weakness, and a rapid pulse. Describe the steps for treating this type of emergency.

CASE STUDY: HYPERTHERMIA AT A STRUCTURE FIRE

▼

Read the scenario and answer the questions that follow. Bear in mind that hyperthermic emergencies can happen even to healthy, fit patients.

You have responded to the scene of a structure fire. It is a hot day, and firefighters are battling a blaze that has fully engulfed a two-story home. You report to the incident commander who points you to a firefighter who is sitting on the tailboard of one of the fire engines. He has stripped off his turnout jacket and helmet and appears somewhat dazed.

"How are you doing?" you ask the firefighter.

He stares at you blankly for a moment. "Fine. I'm just fine." He appears quite hot.

"How about if I just check you out. Your captain seems to think you may have gotten too hot."

"No, I'm fine, really. I just need to sit for a minute. That's all."

23. How should you respond to the firefighter at this point? Why?

24. When you examine the firefighter, you find that he is very hot to the touch, with respirations of 36, strong pulse of 120, and blood pressure at 92/76. As you complete your exam, he vomits. As you continue to talk to him, he becomes more confused. What do you suspect this patient to be suffering from?

25. Another firefighter looks at your patient and states, "Get Frank some water. He looks like he could drink a gallon." Do you agree with this request? Disagree? Explain your answer.

26. List your treatment steps for this patient.

CHAPTER 15

BITES AND STINGS

KEY IDEAS

This chapter focuses on describing the signs, symptoms, and emergency care for poisonous and nonpoisonous snake, insect, spider, and scorpion bites, insect stings, and poisoning by common marine life. Key ideas include the following:

- Poisonous snakebites are considered medical emergencies. Only about one-third of all bites manifest symptoms. When symptoms do develop, they develop quickly.

- Priorities in treating snakebites and other venomous bites and stings focus on supporting the patient's ABCs, limiting the spread of the venom, and arranging for transport without delay.

- In most cases, insect bites and stings can be treated by removing the stinger, cleaning the wound thoroughly, and applying cold to the site to reduce inflammation and pain.

- Emergency care of venomous marine animal bites and stings focuses on slowing the spread of the toxin, removing any stingers or barbs, irrigating and washing the wound, and applying heat to deactivate the toxin.

CONTENT REVIEW

▼

1. You are called to a snakebite incident. As you pull up near the residence, you spot an older man waving you down. As you prepare to exit your vehicle, what is your first priority?
   a. assure scene safety
   b. perform an initial assessment
   c. identify the mechanism of injury
   d. form a general impression of the patient

2. You are called to a bite or sting emergency. To protect your own safety and the safety of others at the scene, what questions related to safety should you consider? Write three examples.

   a.

   b.

   c.

3. A rapidly developing, life-threatening condition that results from an allergic reaction to a bite or sting is called:
   a. anaphylactic shock.
   b. shortness of breath.
   c. altered mental status.
   d. automated defibrillation.

4. Write the general, non–life-threatening signs and symptoms of bites and stings.

5. List the respiratory signs and symptoms of an allergic reaction to a bite or sting.

6. General guidelines for the emergency care of a patient with a bite or sting include the following steps. Write 1–7 to show the correct order in which they should be performed.

_____ **a.** Apply a cold pack to the wound site.

_____ **b.** If a stinger is present in the wound, remove it.

_____ **c.** If breathing is adequate, administer oxygen.

_____ **d.** Inspect the bite or sting site.

_____ **e.** Perform an initial assessment, and treat all life threats.

_____ **f.** Position the injured limb, and manually stabilize it.

_____ **g.** Wash the area around the bite or sting.

7. You should position the site of a bite or sting _____ the level of the patient's heart.
a. slightly above
b. slightly below
c. to the right of
d. to the left of

8. If at any time during the emergency care of a patient who has been bitten or stung you suspect an allergic reaction, you should _____ immediately.
a. inform EMS dispatch
b. apply cold compresses
c. immobilize the extremity
d. apply a constricting band

9. Your patient has had a venomous snakebite to her arm. The bite occurred about 5 minutes ago, and now the bitten area is swollen, red, and quite painful. Your patient is extremely agitated, crying, and shaking. Which of the following should be your next action?
a. As you perform an initial assessment, calm the patient, instruct her to lie still, and position her arm below the level of her heart.
b. Wipe the affected area with alcohol, peroxide, or other mild antiseptic.
c. Place a constricting band above the bite.
d. Suction the bite using an approved suction device.

10. A constricting band should be applied no more than _____ minutes after the patient was bitten by a snake.
a. 10
b. 30
c. 50
d. 70

11. Apply a constricting band _____ inch(es) above the site of the snakebite.
    a. 0 to 1
    b. 2 to 4
    c. 6 to 8
    d. 8 to 12

12. Identify all the characteristics below that indicate a snake may be poisonous.
    a. small, sharp teeth
    b. two large, hollow fangs
    c. pits between its eyes and mouth
    d. triangular head larger than its neck
    e. shapes on a background of white skin

13. Match the characteristics of the bite from a coral snake, a pit-viper, and a nonvenomous snake.

    Pit viper •   • Two large, hollow fangs

                                   • Elliptical pupils

    Nonvenomous snake •   • Pit between eyes and mouth

                                   • Small teeth

    Coral snake •   • Round pupils

14. Critique the following quotes. Write "agree" or "disagree" after each one. If you disagree, write your reasons.

    a. "This guy was just bitten by a rattlesnake. See if you can get some ice cubes, and we'll ice down the bite."

    b. "It's been about 35 minutes or so since John was bitten by that diamondback rattler. We won't need the suction kit. Let's keep him calm, keep the limb stabilized, and get him to the hospital."

    c. "The constricting band needs to be tighter. I can still feel a radial pulse at the wrist."

15. Which one of the following treatments should NOT be performed on a patient who has received a coral-snake bite?
    a. suctioning debris and excess fluids from the airway
    b. administering 100% oxygen by way of nonrebreather mask
    c. mouth-to-mask ventilation with supplemental oxygen
    d. suctioning venom from the bite with an extractor

16. Match the following with the statements that best describe the signs and symptoms that result from their bites or stings.

tick   stingray   tarantula
mite   scorpion   black widow spider
bee   fire ant   brown recluse spider

_____ **a.** Its bite causes pain and spasm in the large muscle groups, leading to respiratory failure and death.

_____ **b.** Its bite causes intense itching, with the site often enlarging to form nodes lasting two or three weeks.

_____ **c.** Its sting is potentially fatal, usually occurs on victim's hands, and leads to drooling, poor coordination, incontinence, and seizures.

_____ **d.** It bites and stings downward as it pivots, producing extremely painful fluid-filled vesicles.

_____ **e.** Its bite can lead to a large ulceration, fever, joint pain, nausea, vomiting, and chills.

_____ **f.** Unlike the black widow, this spider bite causes only moderate pain; other symptoms are very rare.

_____ **g.** An allergic reaction—sometimes severe—to this "garden variety" insect's sting is not uncommon.

_____ **h.** Its bite can lead to Rocky Mountain spotted fever, Lyme disease, and other serious bacterial problems.

_____ **i.** It can leave a painful spine embedded in the patient's skin that should be stabilized in place before transport.

17. You have just returned home from a day-long hike in the woods with several of your friends. When one of them removes his shirt, you see that a tick has attached itself to his belly. To remove it you should:

18. Your 8-year-old son has just been bitten by a yellow jacket. After your initial assessment, you remove the stinger. Explain how.

19. The venom sac attached to a bee stinger can continue to secrete venom into the skin for up to _____ minutes.
  a. 5
  b. 10
  c. 15
  d. 20

CASE STUDY:
BACK-COUNTRY SNAKEBITE
▼

Read the scenario and answer the questions that follow. Be careful to assess the patient's status when trying to decide which interventions would be most helpful. Think about early vs. late signs of pit-viper envenomation, and how these signs may progress as the patient worsens.

You are out on horseback patrolling a hiking area in a mountainous region. You carry a First Responder bag equipped with bandaging materials, manual suction, airway devices, BVM, a small oxygen tank, and a radio. You are about 15 miles from the main campground and ranger station. As you round the bend on a hiking trail, you come upon a frantic scene. Two exhausted hikers are stumbling along, carrying a third hiker who appears disoriented. They spot you and scream, "Quick! Jack's been bitten by a rattlesnake! He's bad! You've got to help us!"

You quickly dismount and help them carry Jack to a shady spot. "Jack was bouldering with us, and he was bitten by a small rattlesnake about an hour ago," explains one of Jack's friends. Jack's hand is swollen and discolored and has two puncture marks on the back. Jack appears pale and sweaty. He responds to you verbally, but seems confused and dazed.

20. Your first action should be to:
  a. apply a constricting band to Jack's arm.
  b. suction the wound to remove any remaining venom.
  c. report to dispatch and request transport for Jack.
  d. administer oxygen to Jack via nonrebreather mask.

21. You further assess Jack and find that his radial pulses are very weak and rapid. He is breathing 36 times per minute. He has vomited twice, according to his friends, and has retched several times since you began emergency care. The correct position in which to place Jack is:
    a. supine with legs elevated.
    b. sitting up with legs dangling.
    c. recovery position (left lateral).
    d. a position of comfort.

22. Your dispatcher is checking into the availability of a helicopter. The trail to the station is wide enough for a ranger vehicle, but it is quite bumpy. If available, the advanced life support helicopter is about 20 minutes of flight time to you and another 20 minutes of flight time back to the hospital. How do you want to evacuate Jack? Set out a plan for evacuating him, taking into account contingency plans if one form of transportation fails.

23. Jack's level of responsiveness begins to drop further. He is now responsive only to painful stimuli. His vital signs are pulse 136, respirations 8, BP 76/44. Describe your plan for treating Jack. Do you want to ventilate him with a BVM? Continue high-flow oxygen via nonrebreather mask? Attempt to insert an NPA or OPA? Explain.

CHAPTER 16

PSYCHOLOGICAL EMERGENCIES AND CRISIS INTERVENTION

KEY IDEAS
▼

This chapter provides an overview of emergency care for patients who are having behavioral and psychological emergencies. It includes discussion about drug and alcohol emergencies, as well as rape and sexual assault. Key ideas include the following:

• In emergencies of any kind, the people involved are susceptible to emotional injury. A behavioral emergency is one in which a patient exhibits "abnormal" behavior, or behavior that is unacceptable or intolerable to the patient, family, or community.

• A behavioral emergency may be the result of a physical illness or injury.

• Psychological care of patients means that you are accepting and helpful, not critical or judgmental.

• Assessing your patient for a possible behavioral emergency should be part of any scene size-up.

• Because signs and symptoms vary so widely and are so similar to many medical conditions, the most reliable indications of a drug- or alcohol-related emergency are likely to come from the scene and the patient history.

• Patients who are suffering from an alcohol or drug overdose are a high priority for transport to a hospital.

• Rape and sexual assault involve both emotional and physical trauma, as well as significant legal issues. When you care for such a patient, remember that his or her coping system has already been stressed to the limit by the attack. Supporting the patient is of critical importance.

CONTENT REVIEW

▼

1. A behavioral emergency may best be defined as one in which a patient exhibits _____ behavior that is _____ to the patient, family, or community.
   a. abnormal, unacceptable
   b. normal, unacceptable
   c. unacceptable, normal
   d. acceptable, normal

2. List 10 factors that can cause a change in a patient's behavior.

   a.

   b.

   c.

   d.

   e.

   f.

   g.

   h.

   i.

   j.

3. You are managing an extremely ill four-year-old who had a seizure at home and now appears to be unresponsive. She has been running a high fever for the past three days. Her parents are very anxious. They demand that you immediately take their child to the hospital. When you tell them that you are waiting for the ambulance to arrive, they begin screaming at you, saying that you are incompetent and that if anything happens to their daughter, you will be held personally responsible.

   a. Are these parents having a behavioral emergency? Explain.

b. Describe an effective strategy for dealing with these parents.

4. List five findings that may indicate that your patient's apparent psychological disturbance is actually being caused by a physical illness or injury.

a.

b.

c.

d.

e.

5. Read the following quotes. Write whether you "agree" or "disagree" with the way in which the First Responder deals with a patient having a behavioral emergency. If you disagree, explain your answer.

a. "Look, pal, I know that you're upset, but killing yourself over a bad relationship is not the answer. Buddy, there's always gonna be other opportunities out there. Keep your chin up."

b. "Look, I realize that you don't think your neck is hurt. However, you need to let me check you out now. Your neck could be broken. Do you want to spend the rest of your life in a wheelchair? I'm here to help you. Don't you want help?"

c. "Paul, I have to tell you that we will be taking you to the hospital for an evaluation. You tried to hurt yourself tonight and we need to make sure you stay safe. I understand that you disagree with us, but we agree with the police officers, and they've decided you need to go."

d. "Trish, my name is Scott. I'm a volunteer with the local fire department. I'm just here to make sure you're okay. Do you want to talk about what happened? Did somebody hurt you? . . . Sure, I can understand that you don't want to talk about it, Trish. Can you tell me if you are hurt anywhere?"

e. "Look, Pat, we all get mad at stuff that goes wrong in our lives. But I'm pretty sure most of us wouldn't consider busting our hand through a plate glass window just because our kids forgot to pick up cat food at the store. You need to sort of stand back and take a look at what you've done, I think."

Questions 6, 7, and 8 may have more than one correct answer. Circle the letters next to all statements that seem correct for each question.

6. You are dealing with a patient who has a life-threatening problem and who is refusing care. What should you do?
   a. Restrain the patient and provide life-saving care.
   b. Inform the patient of the risks of refusing care.
   c. Adequately document the patient's refusal of care.
   d. Attempt to find out why the patient is refusing care.

7. Which two of the following First Responder quotes represent an effective means of managing a patient who has stated, "I just want to kill myself."
   a. "You don't really want to kill yourself. There's so much to live for. Can't you focus on all the good things in your life?"
   b. "You've obviously given up on yourself. What's happened to you? Don't you care how you affect others? Don't you understand that suicide is forever?"
   c. "I need to know. Are you really planning to kill yourself tonight?"
   d. "Have you decided how you would kill yourself?"

8. You have arrived at the residence of a patient with a history of mental illness. His girlfriend meets you out front and tells you that "he's pretty worked up" and that he may have a weapon ("a knife or club or something"). Which two of the following would be correct responses?
   a. Wait outside the residence and call for law enforcement to respond.
   b. Do not allow the woman to reenter the house.
   c. Discreetly investigate to verify the status of the patient.
   d. Call out to the patient from a distance to verify his status.

9. The term "reasonable force" refers to the amount of force needed to:
   a. provide life-saving care.
   b. immobilize a threatening patient.
   c. restrain a patient with metal cuffs.
   d. keep a patient from injuring anyone.

10. The amount of force you use depends on four factors. List them.

    a.

    b.

    c.

    d.

11. The law expects the amount of force you use on a patient to be the same, whether the patient is huddling quietly in a corner or loudly threatening you.

    _____ True

    _____ False

12. One way to protect yourself against false accusations by a patient is to carefully and completely document everything that occurs during a call.

    _____ True

    _____ False

13. The self-administration of one or more drugs in a way that is not in accord with approved medical or social practice is called:
   a. overdose.
   b. drug abuse.
   c. withdrawal.
   d. alcoholism.

14. The effects on the body that occur after a period of abstinence from the drugs or alcohol to which the body has become accustomed are called:
   a. overdose.
   b. drug abuse.
   c. withdrawal.
   d. alcoholism.

15. A(n) _____ emergency is one that involves poisoning by drugs or alcohol.
   a. overdose
   b. drug abuse
   c. withdrawal
   d. alcoholism

16. List four common signs and symptoms of a life-threatening drug- or alcohol-related emergency.

   a.

   b.

   c.

   d.

17. Your patient is unresponsive. You suspect this is a drug- or alcohol-related emergency. To confirm your suspicions, what should you do immediately after your initial assessment?

18. During a drug- or alcohol-related emergency, your immediate goals are to:

a.

b.

c.

19. Which two of the following would be appropriate actions when managing a female patient who was raped and who states that she has no major vaginal or anal injuries?
   a. Complete a careful exam of the vagina and anus to rule out significant bleeding and trauma.
   b. Inform the patient of the steps to be taken between now and her arrival at the hospital.
   c. Allow the patient to wash her hands, arms, and face, but not her genitals.
   d. Perform an initial assessment and a quick, head-to-toe exam to rule out any major trauma.

CASE STUDY: AN ALLEYWAY RAPE AND ASSAULT

▼

Read the case study and answer the questions that follow. Remember that managing a patient can mean managing the patient's emotions as well as actual physical injuries.

It is nearly midnight on a Saturday night, and you have responded to a possible assault victim in an alleyway behind a seedy motel. Dispatch informs you that it may be a stabbing and assault. You arrive to find the scene chaotic. Police officers are everywhere.

You check in with the incident commander and she tells you that your patient is a 27-year-old female who apparently met a drug dealer at the motel to purchase drugs. Instead, the dealer dragged her into the alley, raped her, and then stabbed her. He was frightened off by the motel manager, who had heard the commotion in the alley and came to investigate.

You approach the patient, who sits huddled with a blanket wrapped around her shoulders. She is crying softly, and sits clutching herself.

20. As a First Responder, what would you say to this patient initially? Write out a few sentences.

21. Your patient, Rachel, tells you that she was stabbed once in the upper arm, "pushed around some," and raped. Her skin appears pale, warm, and dry. Her heart rate is 88. How would you proceed with your physical exam of this patient. Why?

22. You delegate the treatment of Rachel's arm laceration to a male First Responder. As he moves to touch the wound with some dressings, she pulls away sharply, clutching herself harder and shouting, "Don't get near me! Don't touch me!" The First Responder pulls away in alarm. How would you deal with her response? Describe at least two strategies for handling this situation.

23. Aside from the knife wound and a few minor bumps and bruises, the patient does not appear to have any significant physical injuries. Blood loss from her stab wound is minor overall. The patient states that she does not have any major vaginal bleeding. What is your treatment plan for this patient at this point? Be specific.

CHAPTER 17

BLEEDING AND SHOCK

KEY IDEAS

This chapter focuses on how to control both external and internal bleeding and how to recognize and manage shock. Key ideas include the following:

- Treating life-threatening bleeding takes priority over all other treatments except emergency care of the patient's airway and breathing.

- Emergency medical care of a patient who has external bleeding includes direct pressure, elevation, and the use of pressure points.

- Internal bleeding is managed by maintaining the patient's ABCs and treating for shock.

- Shock, or hypoperfusion, is a condition that results from the inadequate delivery of oxygenated blood to the body's cells.

- Shock may progress in stages from compensatory shock to decompensated shock to irreversible shock, which is fatal.

- The key to effective prehospital care of the shock patient is early recognition, immediate treatment, and rapid transport to an emergency department.

CONTENT REVIEW

1. When managing an agitated patient with a profusely bleeding head laceration, which of the following describes adequate BSI precautions?
   a. gloves and eye protection
   b. gloves only
   c. gloves and a gown
   d. gloves, gown, and eye protection

2. List the three basic steps for controlling bleeding in order of preference.

   a.

   b.

   c.

3. Pressure should be held at a pulse point until:
   a. the bleeding stops.
   b. a tourniquet can be applied.
   c. bleeding slows to an acceptable rate.
   d. other responders arrive to take over care.

4. Which pressure points are most commonly used to control bleeding?
   a. brachial, femoral
   b. ulnar, carotid
   c. brachial, radial
   d. femoral, pedal

5. Which one of the following statements about tourniquets is NOT true?
   a. A tourniquet can be improvised from a scarf, towel, belt, or necktie.
   b. A tourniquet can completely shut off the blood supply to a limb, causing permanent disability or even loss of the limb.
   c. A tourniquet can be released once bleeding has been controlled.
   d. A tourniquet should be used only as a last resort after all other methods of bleeding control have failed.

6. Match the arterial pulse point with the body part on which it is found.

   dorsalis pedis pulse •   • wrist

   radial pulse •   • top of foot

   femoral pulse •   • groin

   posterior tibial pulse •   • upper arm

   brachial pulse •   • side of ankle

7. An arterial pulse point is a place where:
   a. the blood pressure drops low enough for bleeding to stop.
   b. an artery is protected on all sides by bone and muscle.
   c. an artery is close to a bone and the surface of the skin.
   d. nerve fibers and blood vessels run closely together.

8. The best position for a patient with a nosebleed is:
   a. lying face up with the head tilted back.
   b. sitting up with the head tilted back.
   c. lying on the right or left side.
   d. sitting up and leaning forward.

9. Perfusion is the process by which:
   a. oxygen-carrying red blood cells are created.
   b. cells receive oxygen and have wastes removed.
   c. blood begins to clot when bleeding occurs.
   d. cells break down nutrients to make food.

10. List five signs and symptoms of internal bleeding.

    a.

    b.

    c.

    d.

    e.

11. Patients with some bleeding injuries require oxygen therapy in order to:
    a. increase cellular perfusion.
    b. decrease cellular migration.
    c. increase compensatory shock.
    d. decrease spontaneous clotting.

12. A fellow First Responder has approached you looking for some advice. Here is her story:

    "I just helped the EMTs transport a young guy who ran his car into a telephone pole. His car was a real mess. It took us about 20 minutes to cut him out of it. He had some lacerations from all the broken glass and metal. In fact, I helped to control bleeding to his right forearm. He also said that he had neck and back pain.

    Initially he looked pretty good. The weird thing was that by the time we got him extricated, he was as white as a sheet. After we immobilized him on a long backboard and loaded him in the back of the ambulance, he was breathing really fast and getting combative. The EMT was unable to get a blood pressure, and his pulse was almost too fast to count.

As we transported him with lights and siren, we applied 100% oxygen and elevated his legs. We frantically looked for any signs of trauma, but except for the lacerations and some abdominal pain, we couldn't find anything. The guy died in the ER. What do you think happened? Did we miss something?"

What happened to this patient?

13. Identify all the signs of compensatory shock listed below.
    a. mottled skin
    b. unresponsiveness
    c. normal blood pressure
    d. slightly elevated pulse rates

14. Identify all the signs of decompensated shock listed below.
    a. extreme thirst
    b. very rapid heart rates
    c. normal blood pressures
    d. major changes in mental status

15. Which two of the following statements are true about irreversible shock?
    a. It can be stopped with aggressive treatment.
    b. It leads to the destruction of major organs.
    c. It causes slightly narrowed pulse pressures.
    d. It shunts blood away from the liver and kidneys.

16. The body compensates for losing a lot of blood by shunting blood from the ＿＿＿ to the ＿＿＿ .
    a. liver and kidneys, pancreas and spleen
    b. skin and extremities, major organs
    c. major organs, skin and extremities
    d. major organs, liver and kidneys

17. Which of the following is a late sign of shock?
    a. pale skin
    b. low blood pressure
    c. skin color changes
    d. restlessness or anxiety

18. Which of the following would be among the earliest signs and symptoms of shock?
    a. cool, moist skin
    b. low blood pressure
    c. very rapid heart rate
    d. restlessness or anxiety

19. The _____ the time before symptoms appear in anaphylactic shock, the _____ the risk of a fatal reaction.
    a. greater, shorter
    b. shorter, shorter
    c. shorter, greater
    d. greater, greater

20. Common signs and symptoms of anaphylactic shock include:
    a. fever accompanied by aches and chills.
    b. itching, swelling, and difficulty breathing.
    c. crushing chest pain with shortness of breath.
    d. paralysis of the legs and slow, bounding pulse.

21. The first treatment step in managing shock is to:
    a. keep the patient warm.
    b. assure an open airway.
    c. stop all major bleeding.
    d. loosen restrictive clothing.

Questions 22–26 refer to a 12-year-old female named Paula, who tried to ride her bike through an intersection and was struck by a car traveling 30 mph. She was thrown 25 feet onto concrete pavement.

22. You find Paula in the middle of the intersection, surrounded by Good Samaritans. She appears to be unconscious. What will be your first action at this scene?
    a. Assess Paula's ABCs.
    b. Assess Paula for major injuries.
    c. Make sure that the scene is safe.
    d. Move the Good Samaritans away from Paula.

23. As you complete your initial assessment of Paula, you notice that she has snoring respirations at a rate of six breaths per minute. You also notice that she is bleeding profusely from a large gash just below her left groin. Your next action would be to:
    a. provide mouth-to-mask ventilation to Paula.
    b. open her airway using a jaw-thrust maneuver.
    c. open her airway using a head-tilt/chin-lift maneuver.
    d. apply direct pressure and elevation to the injured leg.

24. Which bleeding control measures would be most appropriate for this patient?
    a. direct pressure and tourniquet
    b. direct pressure and pressure point
    c. direct pressure and elevation
    d. elevation and pressure point

25. You have completed your initial assessment and have performed a quick head-to-toe exam. You found the following: Paula is responsive to pain only. She has a large bruise to her forehead, large scrapes to her left side, a laceration to her leg, and a painful, swollen, deformed right arm. Her vitals are: respirations 6, pulse 120, BP 116/72, with pale, cool, moist skin. Which two of the above findings concern you the most? Why?

26. The following is a list of tasks you complete while managing Paula. Write whether each one is a "high" or "low" priority.

_____ **a.** Maintain Paula's airway using an appropriate airway maneuver.

_____ **b.** Ventilate Paula with supplemental oxygen.

_____ **c.** Try to determine Paula's previous medical history.

_____ **d.** Cover Paula's cuts and bruises.

_____ **e.** Determine if any on-scene bystanders witnessed the incident.

_____ **f.** Establish that the scene is safe from hazards.

_____ **g.** Place an ice pack on Paula's forehead bruise.

_____ **h.** Reassess Paula's level of responsiveness every five minutes.

_____ **i.** Inform bystanders of Paula's condition.

_____ **j.** Determine the speed of the car that struck Paula.

CASE STUDY:
TROUBLE WITH BEES

Read this case study and answer the questions that follow. Focus on the early recognition of shock and the appropriate assessment and treatment of a shock patient. Remember the patient's "Golden Hour"!

It's a sunny day at the park, and you are enjoying a day off the rescue unit with your family. You have just gotten down to a picnic lunch when you hear a commotion at the tables next to yours. There is screaming and shouting and a voice crying out, "Dad, I've been stung by a bee!"

You trot over to investigate, and this is the scene before you: a 10-year-old girl is frantically trying to scrape the stinger of a bee from her shoulder blade, while her father is dumping the contents of the picnic basket out onto the ground. "Where's your bee-sting kit?" he yells. "I can't find it!" The girl is too busy to answer. Her father turns to you. "Please help! I can't find Annie's allergy kit, and she has terrible allergic reactions to bee stings!"

27. Your first action should be to:
    a. have emergency crews dispatched.
    b. assist Annie with scraping off the bee stinger.
    c. assess Annie's airway, breathing, and circulation.
    d. help Annie's father find her allergy kit.

28. Which three body systems might be affected by Annie's allergic reaction?

    a.

    b.

    c.

29. Annie is very agitated. She is jumping up and down, crying, and screaming, "Help me!" What should your response be?

30. Describe your initial assessment of Annie by writing the signs and symptoms of anaphylaxis that you would be watching for.

As you complete your assessment, Annie begins to complain that she can't breathe and that she feels dizzy. Her face and chest are quite flushed, and she is audibly wheezing. She remains conscious but is tiring rapidly. She is breathing 40 times per minute. Her pulse is rapid and weak at the wrist. The on-duty First Responder crew arrives. You call out to them from the picnic bench and turn back to find that Annie is now slumped over and unresponsive.

31. What should your first action be?

32. Given Annie's status, how would you open her airway?

_____ Perform a head-tilt/chin-lift maneuver.

_____ Perform the jaw-thrust maneuver.

As you assist Annie's airway, breathing, and circulation, her father rushes up to you and states that he has found Annie's allergy medicines. He reaches for her arm, and one of the First Responders grabs it. He states, "Hold off giving her any medicine now. The paramedics are only a few minutes away, and they carry medicine for allergy attacks."

33. Do you agree or disagree with this decision? Explain.

CHAPTER 18

SOFT-TISSUE INJURIES

KEY IDEAS

▼

This chapter focuses on the assessment and management of wounds. Key ideas include the following:

- Wounds are classified as open or closed, single or multiple. They are also classified by location.

- Closed wounds include contusions, clamping injuries, and crushing injuries. Open wounds include abrasions, lacerations, penetration/puncture wounds, as well as avulsions, amputations, and crush injuries.

- In general, emergency care of soft-tissue injuries includes treatment for external and internal bleeding.

- Certain open injuries need special consideration during emergency care:
  - The care for penetrating chest injuries, large open neck wounds, and eviscerations usually involves the application of occlusive dressings.
  - An object embedded in an open wound must be stabilized in place (unless it is in the patient's cheek, and then it may be removed).
  - In an amputation, both the patient and the amputated part must be given emergency care.
  - In an avulsion, emergency care includes making sure the flap is lying flat and aligned in its normal position.
  - Open wounds caused by bites should be washed before bandaging.
  - Report the bite incident as per local protocol.

- The basic purposes of dressings and bandages are to control bleeding, to prevent further contamination and damage to the wound, to keep the wound dry, and to immobilize the wound site.

1. Complete the crossword puzzle below.

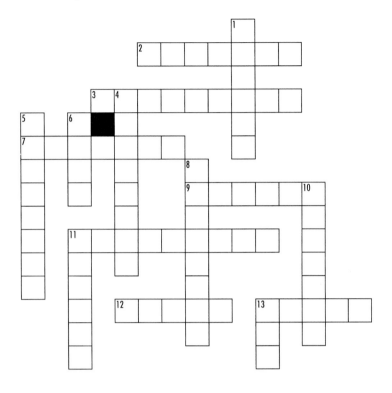

ACROSS

2. A(n) _____ object is one that is embedded in an open wound.
3. A special type of dressing used to form an air-tight seal
7. Used to hold a dressing in place, create pressure, or provide support
9. A viral infection usually associated with animal bites
11. A closed soft-tissue injury characterized by swelling and pain at the injury site
12. A soft-tissue injury is also called a _____ .
13. A(n) _____ dressing is a large, thick, layered pad.

DOWN

1. A hematoma is evident as a lump with _____ discoloration.
4. A(n) _____ injury is one that usually involves a finger or limb stuck in an area smaller than itself.
5. An open wound caused by scraping, rubbing, or shearing away of the epidermis
6. Use a square _____ to tie a bandage in place.
8. A sterile covering for an open wound
10. The state of being free of all microorganisms and spores
11. A triangular bandage that has been folded
13. Take _____ precautions to prevent contact with a patient's blood or body fluids.

2. Identify all the actions listed below that are appropriate for a patient whose finger is stuck in a ring.

   a. Lubricate the finger in order to remove the ring.
   b. Apply a cold pack to the finger to reduce swelling.
   c. Elevate the injured part above the level of the heart.
   d. Heat the ring slightly to expand and loosen it.

3. Your patient has just been struck in the forearm by a baseball bat. Describe what the contusion might look like and how you would care for this injury.

4. Following is a quote from a First Responder describing a patient in a vehicle collision: "We knew by looking at the bent steering column that this guy could have severe blunt trauma, so we immediately treated him for internal bleeding and shock. But it was weird. He initially looked so good. Some abdominal pain, yes, but his skin signs were great, he had a strong radial pulse, and good mental status. During the ongoing assessment, though, we found that he had really decompensated."

   a. What does the First Responder mean when she says that the patient "really decompensated"?

   b. How would the heart rate, blood pressure, mental status, and skin signs of a "decompensated" patient change?

5. Next to each mechanism of injury below, write the type of soft-tissue injury you would expect to see.

avulsion   amputation   puncture/penetration
laceration   bite   abrasion

_____ **a.** Patient was thrown from her bicycle and slid across the pavement.

_____ **b.** Patient's wound occurred when his arm slid along the jagged metal of the car frame.

_____ **c.** Patient suffered an injury when she stepped on a nail.

_____ **d.** Headliner of a car caught the patient's forehead as he was ejected.

_____ **e.** Toddler came screaming from the sandbox, "Fido hurt me!"

_____ **f.** A gang member said that he was cut with a razor blade.

_____ **g.** Police officers state that the assault victim was attacked with a broken whiskey bottle.

_____ **h.** Witnesses think the patient's finger was caught in the power planer.

_____ **i.** Small power sander shot a large splinter of wood at patient's arm.

6. Identify all of the following soft-tissue injuries that carry a high risk of infection.
   a. abrasion
   b. laceration
   c. puncture
   d. human bite

7. Lacerations can cause which one or more of the following problems? (There is more than one answer.)
   a. infection
   b. permanent scarring
   c. cut tendons or nerves
   d. severe, uncontrolled bleeding

8. List three factors that influence the severity of a stab wound.

   a.

   b.

   c.

9. Control of bleeding from an amputation should first be attempted using:
   a. a splint.
   b. a tourniquet.
   c. pressure points.
   d. direct pressure and elevation.

10. The steps below describe how to manage a patient with an amputation of the forearm. Write 1–10 to put the steps in the correct order.

   _____ a. Remove clothing to expose the entire injury site.

   _____ b. Wrap the severed part in saline-moistened, sterile gauze.

   _____ c. Dress and bandage the stump.

   _____ d. Administer oxygen by way of a nonrebreather mask.

   _____ e. Assure an open airway and adequate breathing.

   _____ f. Complete an initial assessment.

   _____ g. Control bleeding with direct pressure and elevation.

   _____ h. Size up the scene for hazards and the mechanism of injury.

   _____ i. Wipe away loose particles of foreign matter from the wound.

   _____ j. Perform an ongoing assessment until the EMTs arrive to take over care.

11. List four questions that will help you to better understand the mechanism of injury that has caused a penetrating, crushing, or clamping injury.

   a.

   b.

   c.

   d.

12. Which one of the following crushing-injury sites would most likely result in shock?
   a. radius
   b. humerus
   c. femur
   d. fibula

13. Which one of the following steps should NOT be taken to help a patient with a serious crushing injury?
    a. Administer oxygen by way of nonrebreather mask at 15 lpm.
    b. Elevate the patient's legs about 8 to 12 inches, if appropriate.
    c. Apply a cold pack to the injury site.
    d. Keep the patient warm and quiet.

14. You are at the scene of a stabbing. A fellow First Responder turns to you and states the following: "The patient was stabbed in the back just above the scapula. It looks like there is minimal bleeding from the wound. The police found the knife, and it only has a two-inch blade, so this guy should be okay." Agree? Disagree? Explain.

15. You are caring for a patient who has a one-foot steel rod impaled in his abdomen. Which one of the following would NOT be an appropriate action?
    a. Manually stabilize the steel rod.
    b. Remove clothing to expose the injury site.
    c. Cut the rod to make it easier to manage.
    d. Administer oxygen by way of a nonrebreather mask.

16. Correct treatment for a patient who has a pen impaled through his cheek includes which one of the following?
    a. Stabilize the pen with bulky dressings.
    b. Cut the pen to make it a manageable size.
    c. Position the pen so it cannot occlude the airway.
    d. Remove the pen and apply bulky dressings to the wound.

17. Because significant soft-tissue injuries to the chest can allow air to flow where it should not, apply a(n) _____ dressing to all open chest wounds.
    a. occlusive
    b. pressure
    c. bulky
    d. roller

18. Open soft-tissue injuries to the neck should be sealed airtight with a(n) _____ dressing.
    a. occlusive
    b. pressure
    c. bulky
    d. roller

19. On rare occasions, you may be required to manage an evisceration. Describe how you would dress or bandage it.
    a. Replace exposed organs and cover with a thick, moist dressing.
    b. Replace exposed organs and cover with light, dry gauze.
    c. Leave exposed organs as found and cover with a thick, moist dressing.
    d. Leave exposed organs as found and cover with light, dry gauze.

20. Proper care for a patient with an avulsion to the scalp includes which one of the following?
    a. Place the skin flap in its normal position.
    b. Fold the skin flap away from the open wound.
    c. Dress the wound exactly the way you found it.
    d. Remove the skin flap and place it on a cold pack.

21. Dog bites should include which of the following treatments? (There is more than one answer.)
    a. Check for teeth fragments.
    b. Wash the wound with soap and water.
    c. Apply direct pressure to control bleeding.
    d. Follow local protocols on reporting requirements.

22. One of the primary purposes of a dressing is to:
    a. hold a bandage in place.
    b. prevent the bandage from sticking to the wound.
    c. ensure that the wound remains sterile.
    d. prevent further contamination of the wound.

23. Which one of the following would NOT make a good dressing?
    a. bath towel
    b. handkerchief
    c. toilet tissue
    d. sanitary napkin

24. Which one of the following is an example of an occlusive dressing?
    a. burn pad
    b. gauze pad
    c. ABD dressing
    d. aluminum foil

25. You are caring for a patient with a three-inch laceration to his arm with minimal bleeding. This wound would best be covered with which two of the following?
    a. a burn pad
    b. a bandage compress
    c. a gauze pad
    d. petroleum gauze

26. Which two of the following statements about bandaging are true?
    a. Make sure the bandage is sterile.
    b. Remove a patient's jewelry first.
    c. Bandages should allow air to reach the wound.
    d. Loosen bandaging if it proves to be too tight.

27. Describe four uses of triangular bandages:

a.

b.

c.

d.

28. Self-adhering, form-fitting bandages are known as:
a. cravats.
b. roller bandages.
c. bandage compresses.
d. triangular bandages.

29. Analyze the following statements by First Responders regarding bandaging. Then write "agree" or "disagree" beside each one. If you disagree, explain why.

a. "My patient just told me that the bandage is too tight, but I convinced her to leave it the way it is so that the laceration won't start bleeding again."

b. "The laceration is about four inches long on the side of the patient's foot. It was bleeding pretty badly when I arrived on scene, so I went ahead and covered up the entire foot with bandages."

c. "I thought that the bandage on the forearm wound might be too tight, but the patient said it felt fine. His fingers were warm and pink, and he had a good radial pulse, so I left it."

d. "My partner had covered the wound with some gauze dressings and roller bandages, but the edges of the wound were exposed, so I removed the bandaging and added a larger trauma dressing to cover the entire area."

e. "I made a pressure bandage by applying some dressings to the wound and then folding two triangular bandages into cravats and tying them tightly around the dressings."

30. The saw Ray Gonzalez was using slipped and sliced open his thigh. He sees all the blood and is terrified. "I'm going to die!" he says in a husky whisper. You answer him:
    a. "Most people don't die from cuts like this. Just relax. It'll be okay."
    b. "You're not going to die. Now, if you had gotten cut where your femoral artery is, that would be a different story."
    c. "I'm going to help control the bleeding here. You can help me by lying back down so that I can see where to put my dressings."
    d. "It looks pretty bad, but I'll do what I can to get this bleeding under control."

31. You are still with Ray Gonzalez, the patient described above. You don gloves and then place a handful of 4 × 4 gauze pads on the wound. They are quickly saturated with blood. Which dressing or bandage should you apply next to this wound?
    a. more gauze pads
    b. an occlusive dressing
    c. a roller bandage
    d. a trauma dressing

32. After applying direct pressure with dressings to Mr. Gonzalez's wound for several minutes, it appears that the bleeding has slowed to a trickle. Which of the following bandaging materials would make the best pressure bandage?
    a. cravats
    b. triangular bandages
    c. roller bandages
    d. elastic bandages

33. Mr. Gonzalez has calmed down considerably. He props himself up from his supine position and asks, "Do you think I cut off blood flow to the rest of my leg?" Describe how you would go about determining whether or not there is blood circulating to his lower leg.

CASE STUDY:
CHILD VS. RUSTY PIPE

▼

Read the scenario and answer the questions that follow. Focus on the priorities for managing a soft-tissue injury. Remember your patient assessment plan.

You have just exited a transit bus on your way home from work when you hear screams. You decide which house they are coming from—the Johnsons—and trot over. Along a side walkway is an overturned bicycle and a huge splatter of blood. From the backyard you hear the strangled sobs of a child and the frantic voice of a woman, probably his mother.

You follow the trail of blood to the backyard. "Can I help?" you call out as the mother and child come into view.

"Please, please help! Danny is bleeding badly," answers the child's mother. She has taken the child to a garden hose and is dousing a large, jagged laceration with water. It is still bleeding profusely. "He cut himself on a rusty pipe at the side of the house," she explains. Her four-year-old son is frantic, sobbing, and struggling to free himself from her hold.

34. What should be your first step in getting ready to assist this child?

35. Describe your strategy for helping the child to calm down.

36. You move to turn the hose off. The mother says, "Keep the water on. He cut his leg on a rusty drain spout." What is your response?

37. You finally are able to examine the wound. It is a three-inch-long laceration, about one inch deep, on the front of his thigh. It stretches from midway down his thigh to his knee. Describe the location and extent of the wound. Use three of the following terms: proximal; distal; anterior; posterior; midway.

38. List the steps in controlling bleeding from this injury.

39. You have controlled the child's bleeding and have calmed both him and his mother. Paramedics have just arrived. Give them a patient hand-off report. (Information: you estimate that the child has lost perhaps 200 milliliters of blood.)

CHAPTER 19

INJURIES TO CHEST, ABDOMEN, AND GENITALIA

KEY IDEAS

This chapter describes different types of chest, abdominal, and genital injuries along with appropriate assessment and emergency treatment. Key ideas include the following:

- Chest injuries are serious emergencies that require immediate activation of the EMS system with rapid transport to a trauma center or other medical facility.

- Initial emergency care of chest injuries focuses on maintaining the patient's airway, breathing, and circulation. Additional treatment includes stabilizing flail chests and fractured ribs, and sealing puncture wounds with airtight dressings.

- Injuries to the abdomen can cause bleeding and shock, infection, and internal organ damage. Surgery is usually required to repair major abdominal injuries.

- Field care for abdominal injuries focuses on supporting the patient's airway, breathing, and circulation.

- Care for injuries to the genitalia includes treating for shock and managing the soft-tissue injuries.

CONTENT REVIEW

1. Write five signs and symptoms of chest trauma.

   a.

   b.

   c.

   d.

   e.

2. In general, basic emergency care of a chest injury must include the following steps. Write 1–4 to place them in the correct order.

   _____ a. Perform a quick physical exam.

   _____ b. Control any signs of external bleeding.

   _____ c. Assure adequate ventilations.

   _____ d. Maintain an open airway.

3. Why is the immediate activation of the EMS system an important step in caring for a chest-injured patient?

4. Which one of the following is NOT a sign of a chest injury?
   a. coughing up blood
   b. elevated blood pressure
   c. difficulty breathing
   d. signs of shock

5. The most serious threat posed by injuries to the chest is possible damage to the:
   a. heart and lungs.
   b. stomach and intestinal organs.
   c. intercostal muscles and ribs.
   d. esophagus and ribs.

6. Mechanisms of blunt injury to the chest may include which of the following? (There may be more than one answer.)
   a. being thrown against a steering wheel
   b. arm crushed against the side door in a side-impact collision
   c. primary phase of a blast or explosion
   d. head-first fall of 15 feet or more

7. Why does the victim of traumatic asphyxia have distended neck veins and a swollen appearance of the head, neck, and shoulders?

8. A flail chest occurs when two or more adjacent ribs are broken, each in two or more places.

   _____ True

   _____ False

9. A flail chest may be the result of:
   a. a bruised or perforated lung.
   b. fractures of the sternum, cartilage, or ribs.
   c. a puncture wound to the chest.
   d. a severe tension pneumothorax.

10. When the patient exhales, the flail segment protrudes while the rest of the chest wall contracts. This is called:
    a. a typical guarding position.
    b. a sucking chest wound.
    c. paradoxical breathing.
    d. pneumothorax.

11. Flail chest can lead to immediate life-threatening problems. Identify all those listed below.
    a. hypoxic drive
    b. abdominal evisceration
    c. severed femoral arteries
    d. puncture wounds of the lung
    e. serious bleeding into the thorax
    f. inadequate oxygenation of the heart

12. To stabilize a flail chest:
    a. apply an airtight dressing.
    b. tape a small pillow over the injury site.
    c. place five or six pounds over the flail area.
    d. lay the patient down on the side opposite the flail area.

13. Open chest injuries do not upset the delicate balance of pressure between the inside and outside of the chest.

    _____ True

    _____ False

14. Open injuries to the back are considered open chest injuries.

    _____ True

    _____ False

15. Sometimes an open wound to the chest bubbles or makes a sucking noise. Such a wound is typically called:
    a. grating or crepitus.
    b. tracheal deviation.
    c. sucking chest wound.
    d. bubbling chest wound.

16. Treatment for both an open chest injury and a closed one are basically the same with one very important exception. What is it?

17. Describe how you should apply an occlusive dressing over a sucking chest wound.

18. If you have to improvise an occlusive dressing for an open chest wound, use household _____ but NOT household _____ .
    a. plastic wrap, aluminum foil
    b. paper towels, aluminum foil
    c. aluminum foil, plastic wrap
    d. plastic wrap, paper towels

19. If the patient with an open chest injury develops increased respiratory distress after application of an occlusive dressing, you must:
    a. add another occlusive dressing over the wound site.
    b. tape down the fourth side of the dressing.
    c. use your hand to form a tighter seal.
    d. release the seal immediately.

20. The term "pneumothorax" may be defined as collapse of the lungs caused by blood in the chest.

    _____ True

    _____ False

21. The term "hemothorax" may be defined as collapse of the lungs caused by air in the chest.

    _____ True

    _____ False

22. You are managing a patient who has suffered blunt abdominal injuries after impacting the steering wheel of her car. Describe the types of injuries her liver and her intestines may have incurred.

23. List eight signs and symptoms that would indicate a patient has an abdominal injury.

a.

b.

c.

d.

e.

f.

g.

h.

24. Very briefly describe emergency care of a patient with a closed abdominal injury.

25. Read the following statement: "Our patient was struck in the stomach with a shovel. He has some moderate abdominal pain. All I can see is a small laceration to his abdomen with minimal bleeding, so I don't think he's hurt too badly." Do you agree with this rescuer's comments? Explain.

26. The most comfortable position for a patient with an abdominal injury is:
  a. supine, with the knees flexed.
  b. left lateral recumbent.
  c. sitting up.
  d. prone.

27. Proper care for an abdominal evisceration includes:
  a. positioning the patient on his or her side.
  b. placing a moist, sterile dressing over the evisceration.
  c. gently replacing the eviscerated organs in the abdomen.
  d. covering the eviscerated tissue with plastic wrap.

28. You should maintain the temperature of the area of an abdominal evisceration by covering the dressings with:
  a. a heating pad.
  b. chemical hot packs.
  c. a particle-free towel.
  d. immersion in warm water.

29. Emergency care for a torn or avulsed penis includes all of the following EXCEPT:
  a. wrapping the penis in a moistened, sterile dressing.
  b. removing any penetrating objects.
  c. applying a cold pack to relieve pain and swelling.
  d. controlling bleeding with direct pressure.

30. Which one of the following is NOT a recommended treatment step for injuries to the female genitalia?
  a. Treat the patient for shock.
  b. Control bleeding with direct pressure.
  c. Insert sterile dressings into a bleeding vagina.
  d. Use cold packs over the dressings to relieve pain.

31. You are treating a female sexual assault victim. She has bruises to her arms and neck. She states that she has no vaginal bleeding. She wants to clean herself before going to the hospital. Which two of the following responses would NOT be appropriate for you to make?
  a. "I understand what you've told me, but I still need to check your vagina for injuries."
  b. "Are you hurt anywhere else?"
  c. "It's best that you don't wash up until you've been checked at the hospital."
  d. "Can you tell me specifically what happened so that I can understand where you might be injured?"

32. In the space provided, write the term described by each statement. Some terms will not be used.

liver   spleen   pelvic cavity
guarding   abdominal cavity   thoracic cavity
upper left   upper right   lower right

   a. A solid organ found primarily in the upper right abdominal quadrant is the

     _____ .

   b. An instinctive reaction to protect a painful abdomen is _____ .

   c. A solid organ found in the upper left abdominal quadrant is the

     _____ .

   d. The body cavity that contains organs of digestion and excretion is the

     _____ .

   e. The body cavity that is bounded by the lower part of the spine, the hip bones, and the

     pubis is the _____ .

   f. The kidneys are located in the upper right and the _____
     quadrant of the abdomen.

The next five questions have to do with Dave, a man in his 20s. He rode his motorcycle around a bend at about 40 mph, laid the bike down, and slid into a tree. There was no loss of consciousness, but he is lying on his back with his knees drawn up. He still has on a full set of riding leathers, but bystanders have removed his full-face helmet.

33. Your first step in emergency care of Dave should be to:
   a. give Dave high-flow oxygen.
   b. assess Dave's abdomen and pelvis.
   c. maintain manual immobilization of his spine.
   d. check Dave's airway, respirations, and pulses.

34. Dave appears to be alert and oriented but in a lot of pain. You find that his respirations are 26, his pulse is 120, and his blood pressure is 134/78. His skin is pale, warm, and slightly moist. These findings suggest that Dave may be experiencing:
   a. progressive shock.
   b. compensatory shock.
   c. irreversible shock.
   d. latent shock.

35. Number the following steps 1–7 to show the order in which they should be performed.

_____ **a.** Introduce yourself to Dave and quickly assess his level of responsiveness and chief complaint.

_____ **b.** Perform a head-to-toe physical exam, in particular palpating Dave's abdomen and pelvis to assess injury.

_____ **c.** Ask your partner to maintain manual stabilization of Dave's head and neck.

_____ **d.** Apply high-concentration oxygen via nonrebreather mask.

_____ **e.** Check Dave's airway, breathing, and circulation.

_____ **f.** Size up the scene for dangers and mechanisms of injury.

_____ **g.** Place a gauze bandage over a small laceration you discover on Dave's arm.

36. Write the pertinent questions you would ask when examining Dave's abdomen.

D:

O:

T:

S:

37. From your exam, you find that Dave does NOT have any neck or back pain. Should you maintain manual stabilization of his head and neck? Why or why not?

CASE STUDY: BAR FIGHT

Read this scenario and answer the questions that follow. When reading through the scenario, think about everything you have learned in this course so far.

It's 11 o'clock on a Saturday night, and you respond to reports of an assault at Rudy's Alnight Tavern. You arrive to find the scene secured by local law enforcement. Your patient, a 27-year-old man, is lying on the floor at the back of the bar. A police officer tells you that the patient was apparently attacked by three adult males after an argument broke out at the pool tables. He was thrown to the floor and then kicked and beaten with pool cues. A bloody knife was taken from one of the suspects.

You move to the patient's side and are hit immediately with the heavy smell of beer on his breath. He is clutching his chest, moaning. You can see that he is pale and having a difficult time breathing. Blood is plastered all over his hands and chest.

38. Given the mechanism of injury involved, you expect the patient to be suffering from all of the following EXCEPT:
    a. blunt chest trauma.
    b. penetrating chest injuries.
    c. compression chest injuries.
    d. contusions and lacerations.

39. What information presented so far makes you the most suspicious that this patient may have a serious chest injury?
    a. The police officer reported that the patient was attacked by three adult males.
    b. The mechanisms of injury include pool cues and possibly a knife.
    c. The patient has blood "plastered all over his hands and chest."
    d. The patient appears extremely pale, has some type of chest injury, and is having difficulty breathing.

40. After a scene size-up, which of the following should be your next action?
    a. Perform an initial assessment.
    b. Apply oxygen at 6 lpm by nasal cannula.
    c. Locate the patient's wounds and stop the bleeding.
    d. Remove the patient's clothing to check for hidden injuries.

41. Your physical exam finds bruising to the chest and a three-quarter-inch laceration just below the left nipple. You hear a bubbling noise at the wound site when the patient inhales and exhales. Correct treatment of this injury includes:
    a. immediately covering the wound with any available wrapping.
    b. immediately bandaging the wound with a 4 × 4 and an elastic bandage.
    c. continuing with the physical exam until it is complete.
    d. immediately applying an occlusive dressing, sealed on three sides.

42. After appropriately caring for the sucking chest wound, you notice the patient becoming increasingly anxious, short of breath, and cyanotic. His neck veins are bulging. What's happening to your patient, and what action should you take to correct it?

43. This patient's vital signs initially were: respirations 20, pulse 106, BP 128/76. He is alert and his skin is pink, warm, and moist. You recheck his vital signs five minutes later and find: respirations 36, pulse 144, BP 82/48, confusion (reduced level of responsiveness), and pale, cool, moist skin. Explain why the following vital signs have changed.

Respirations:

Pulse:

BP:

Level of responsiveness:

44. This patient's rapidly deteriorating vital signs indicate he requires immediate transportation to a trauma center. List tasks that you could complete while you wait for transport to arrive.

45. You have treated the patient for his wounds and administered oxygen. Paramedics have just arrived on scene. Write a hand-off report you could give to them about this patient.

CHAPTER 20

BURN EMERGENCIES

KEY IDEAS
▼

This chapter provides an overview of the methods of classifying burns and describes basic emergency care of burns, as well as special types of burn injuries. Key ideas include the following:

- Burns are complex injuries that can impair a number of the body's functions, including fluid balances, body temperature, and joint function.

- The severity of a burn is determined by the depth of the burn, percentage of body surface burned, location of the burn, accompanying complications, and age of the patient.

- Treatment for burns focuses on stopping the source of the burning, maintaining the patient's ABCs, and covering the burned area with sterile dressings.

- Inhalation injuries can cause severe, life-threatening respiratory distress. In addition to respiratory burns, victims of these injuries can be poisoned by the substance that has been inhaled.

- Chemical burns require aggressive irrigation. All significant chemical burns should be treated as severe.

- The most important priority in cases of electrical burns is scene safety. Treatment focuses on maintaining the patient's ABCs and should include spinal immobilization.

CONTENT REVIEW

1. The severity of a burn depends on many factors. List four:

   a.

   b.

   c.

   d.

2. Match the signs and symptoms to the related term.

   charring •   • superficial burns

   red skin and swelling •

   intense pain •   • partial-thickness burns

   red skin and blisters •

   little or no pain •   • full-thickness burns

3. Read each description. Then write whether the burn described is a superficial (S), partial thickness (P), or full thickness (F).

   _____ a. A burn that results in redness and blistering; the epidermis and dermal layers of skin are usually burned

   _____ b. A burn that involves muscle and bone

   _____ c. A burn that appears white, dark, or charred; extends through all dermal layers and can involve subcutaneous layers

   _____ d. A burn that involves the epidermal layer alone

4. You are managing a patient who was burned in a grease fire. He has burns covering his entire anterior chest and abdomen, as well as his anterior left arm. Using the "rule of nines," calculate the percentage of his body that has been burned.

5. Decide if each patient has critical, moderate, or minor burns. Write your answer in the space provided.

   a. A 65-year-old patient received full-thickness burns to her hands and face from hot grease.

   b. A 23-year-old received superficial burns to his abdomen when he spilled a pot of boiling water.

   c. A 16-year-old received partial-thickness burns to her arms and chest from hot oil after her car was hit by a truck. She also suffered a fractured arm and leg.

   d. A 9-year-old was rescued from a burning residence. He has a rasping cough and soot in his nostrils.

   e. A 35-year-old received partial-thickness burns to his left forearm after leaning up against a hot metal surface at work.

   f. A 27-year-old received a superficial burn to the back of her left hand while tending the fire in her wood stove.

   g. A 17-year-old was splashed in the eyes with a mild acid solution in the chemistry lab at school.

6. Why do children under the age of 5 and adults over the age of 55 tolerate burns so poorly?

7. The top priority in managing a burn patient is to:
   a. eliminate the cause of the burn.
   b. determine the severity of the burn.
   c. remove the patient from the source of the burn.
   d. examine the patient for airway and breathing problems.

8. Which one of the following statements regarding the treatment of burns is true?
   a. Ice may be used to cover a burn.
   b. Cover burns with wet, sterile dressings.
   c. Cover burns with dry, sterile dressings.
   d. Grease or fat may be used to cover burns.

9. Chemical burns should be flushed with water for a minimum of _____ minutes.
   a. 5
   b. 10
   c. 15
   d. 20

10. You have responded to a victim of a house fire who has burns and inhalation injuries. The emergency care you need to provide is described below. Number the steps 1–7 to show the correct order in which they should be performed.

   _____ a. Perform an initial assessment.

   _____ b. Determine the history of the burn.

   _____ c. Administer oxygen via nonrebreather mask.

   _____ d. Remove the patient from the source of the burn.

   _____ e. Stop the burning process.

   _____ f. Cover the burns.

   _____ g. Assess the extent and severity of the patient's burns.

11. Identify all the signs and symptoms of smoke inhalation listed below.
   a. cyanosis
   b. noisy breathing
   c. skin rash or hives
   d. shortness of breath
   e. singed nasal hairs
   f. cough or hoarseness
   g. burns to the face
   h. carbon in the sputum
   i. difficulty speaking
   j. restricted chest movement
   k. bruising of the skin
   l. puncture/penetrating wounds
   m. abrasions or lacerations

12. Why is it necessary to constantly reassess a patient who has suffered inhalation injuries?

13. You are managing a patient who received burns to his arms and face following a house fire. Your partner tells you, "Remove everything on his arms and hands so that we can take care of his burns." He has rings on his fingers, a watch on one wrist, and charred clothing hanging from both arms, some of it embedded in the burns. Which of these items do you want to remove? Which do you want to leave alone? Why?

14. You are responding to a car vs. power pole. You arrive to find two uninjured passengers. You note that a power line is draped across their car. There appears to be no immediate fire or explosion danger. One of the occupants is attempting to open a door to get out, but it appears jammed. What should these occupants do, and why?

15. List five signs and symptoms of electrical shock.

a.

b.

c.

d.

e.

16. Care for a patient with lightning burns the same way you would care for any patient with the following two exceptions:

a.

b.

CASE STUDY: ELECTROCUTION VICTIM
▼

Read the scenario and answer the questions that follow. Remember that patients who have been electrocuted may have extensive internal injuries and organ damage not immediately evident. Be sure to prioritize your care to treat the patient for life-threatening injuries first.

You arrive at a canal levy where a farmer was electrocuted by a downed power line. Bystanders tell you that the farmer was driving his tractor near the levy when he ran into a downed power line. He was electrocuted when he hopped off the tractor to investigate.

You see that the farmer is lying near his tractor. Members of the local fire department who arrived on scene before you tell you that they removed the power line and it is safe to approach the patient.

17. As you cautiously move closer to the farmer you notice that the soles of your feet begin to tingle. What is causing this, and what should you do?

18. The scene is now safe. You call to the farmer, but he does not respond. Based on what you know about electrocution injuries, what injuries are you expecting to find, and what equipment will you need to manage these injuries?

19. Where would you expect to find contact burns on this patient, and how will you treat them?

20. Vital signs on this patient are as follows: The farmer is unresponsive, with a pulse of 44 and respirations of 8 per minute. The farmer's blood pressure is unobtainable. You can see an ugly burn on the farmer's foot and both of his legs appear to be fractured. The two fire department crew members are busy securing the scene from curious onlookers. Which of these findings should you manage first? Why?

CHAPTER 21

AGRICULTURAL AND INDUSTRIAL EMERGENCIES

KEY IDEAS

This chapter focuses on injuries that occur in agricultural and industrial settings. Key ideas include the following:

- Farming is a hazardous occupation. The number of deaths in work-related accidents exceeds those occurring in mining, construction, or transportation and public utilities.

- The First Responder care for farm-related injuries is the same as for any other injury. Understanding common mechanisms of injury and the types of farm equipment involved will help the First Responder decide on the best care for patients.

- Farm machinery must be stabilized and shut down before the patient can be assessed and treated.

- Lifting farm equipment off a patient and disentangling a patient requires teamwork, specialized equipment, and training.

- The top priority in responding to any farm or industrial accident is the safety of all responders.

- Industrial accidents may include structural collapses, toxic gas releases, hazardous materials contamination, and entrapment. All of these emergencies require specially trained teams to safely rescue and treat the patient.

CONTENT REVIEW

1. Explain how each of the following factors contributes to the severity of farming-related injuries.

   a. Farm equipment design:

   b. Expense of new equipment:

   c. Time required to disentangle farmers from machinery:

   d. Remoteness of many farms:

2. There are four conditions that must exist before disentanglement and rescue of a patient should begin. Identify them in the list below.
   a. Farm equipment has been stabilized.
   b. There is time for helicopter transport.
   c. The patient has life-threatening injuries.
   d. Hazards, such as leaking fuel, are present.
   e. Farm equipment engines have been shut down.
   f. The patient has been stabilized.
   g. The patient is unresponsive.
   h. Hazards have been controlled.

3. You have responded to a farming accident in which a farmer has caught her hand in a corn picker. When you arrive, her arm is still entangled in the machinery. You note that she is bleeding profusely from the injury. Describe your strategy for controlling bleeding prior to disentanglement.

4. Describe the mechanisms of injury common to tractors and other farm equipment.

    a. Pinch points:

    b. Wrap points:

    c. Shear points:

    d. Crush points:

    e. Stored energy:

5. The most common cause of farm-related fatalities is the:
    a. tractor.
    b. power take-off shaft (PTO).
    c. combine.
    d. auger.

6. Some farm equipment manufacturers use color codes to help operators quickly identify controls. Describe what each color usually represents.

    a. Red:

    b. Yellow:

    c. Black:

7. What is the most common type of fatal injury associated with farm tractors?
   a. compression injury
   b. crushing injury
   c. laceration
   d. wrapping injury

8. The first step in shutting down farm equipment is to stabilize it. Identify all the methods listed below by which this can be done.
   a. Set the parking brakes.
   b. Block or chock the wheels.
   c. Drive it to a flat surface.
   d. Tie the machine to another vehicle.

9. Do not stop patient care during lifting operations. Both efforts should continue at the same time.

   _____ True

   _____ False

10. It is uncommon for patients involved in a tractor rollover to have chemical burns to the eyes.

    _____ True

    _____ False

11. In any emergency involving a tractor rollover, suspect crushing injuries to the patient's head, chest, and abdomen.

    _____ True

    _____ False

12. The best tools for lifting large, irregularly shaped machines such as tractors are:
    a. cribs.
    b. power hydraulic tools.
    c. high-pressure airbags.
    d. cranes or boom trucks.

13. Airbags are most efficient during the first _____ to _____ inches of lift.
    a. 3, 5
    b. 5, 7
    c. 7, 9
    d. 9, 11

14. During any extrication of a patient from farm equipment, two rescuers should take charge. One should direct the lifting from the front and another should direct the effort from the back.

    _____ True

    _____ False

15. You should watch the patient during the lift to make sure that the part to be lifted is moving properly and that another part is not putting more pressure on the patient. If conditions change, you should:
    a. lift the part that is pressing on the patient.
    b. tell the patient that it will all be over soon.
    c. advise the rescuer leading the lifting operation.
    d. take over the leader's job to make sure the patient survives.

16. Which of the following would NOT be an appropriate method of disentangling a patient from a PTO?
    a. Cut the shaft with a power saw.
    b. Run the PTO until the patient is freed.
    c. Cut the patient's clothing with rescue knives.
    d. Uncouple the shaft and transport it with the patient.

17. Combines can cause crushing and amputation injuries when farmers get caught in the machine's:
    a. augers.
    b. roller chains.
    c. sprockets.
    d. belts and pulleys.

18. Which two of the following statements are true of augers?
    a. They are used to move grain from a combine to trucks or wagons.
    b. They often cause amputations and entanglements too severe to be dealt with in the field.
    c. They can be reversed to free an entrapped patient.
    d. They can be cut using a torch.

19. When rescuing a patient from a grain tank, which two of the following directives should you follow?
    a. Wear a disposable mechanical filter respirator.
    b. Use the gravity gate or auger to release the grain.
    c. Cut uniform triangular holes above the level of the grain.
    d. Secure the patient with a lifeline once he or she is exposed.

20. Which of the following signs and symptoms would indicate the patient is suffering from silo gas inhalation? (There may be more than one answer.)
    a. cyanosis
    b. coughing
    c. eye irritation
    d. nausea and vomiting

21. The top two priorities for managing an industrial rescue include which of the following tasks?
    a. Assessing the patient to determine the extent of his or her injuries.
    b. Treating the patient's airway, breathing, and circulation.
    c. Assessing the scene for dangers such as the presence of hazardous materials, structural instability, and the threat of fire.
    d. Determining the type of equipment and number of rescuers necessary to manage the emergency.

CASE STUDY: TRACTOR ROLLOVER

Read this scenario and answer the questions that follow. Focus on managing both the overturned tractor and the patient. Remember that scene safety must be your top priority!

You are the First Responder on the scene of a tractor rollover. The farmer, Mike Stevenson, was working on a steep hillside when his tractor rolled over sideways down the hill. As you pull up to the scene, you see that the tractor has come to rest on its side.

Mike's son, Ted, witnessed the accident and states that the tractor rolled over at least twice. The tractor does have a roll bar, and Ted states that his father is wearing a seat belt. The tractor cab is wedged against the embankment. You are unable to see Mike. The tractor engine is still running.

22. Your first action should be to:
    a. cut the tractor's fuel supply.
    b. determine if Mike is still alive.
    c. stabilize the tractor by setting its parking brake.
    d. call for additional resources to assist with this rescue.

23. The emergency scene is at least an hour's ground-transport time from the closest hospital. You should advise your dispatch center to send which of the following EMS transport teams?
    a. paramedic-staffed ambulance
    b. EMT-staffed ambulance
    c. nurse-staffed helicopter
    d. nurse-staffed helicopter and paramedic-staffed ambulance

24. The safest method for shutting off the tractor engine is to:
    a. cut the fuel line and tie it to another vehicle.
    b. discharge a CO_2 or Halon fire extinguisher into the air intake.
    c. slow the engine with the throttle and switch off the ignition key.
    d. loosen the fuel filter and chock the wheels.

Additional rescue personnel arrive. Nearby farmers arrive with cables and chains and lock up the overturned tractor's rear wheels. The tractor engine is turned off. You climb onto the tractor and find that Mike is still seat-belted into the cab. His right leg is crushed, pinned between the tractor and the embankment. He is crying out in severe pain and appears pale and sweaty. His radial pulse is rapid and weak. He does not appear to have any other major injuries.

You determine that the tractor needs to be lifted about a foot in order to free Mike's leg. Rescue personnel at the scene have arrived with a large boom truck and hand-powered hydraulic jacks. The rescue unit outfitted with high-pressure airbags is 20 to 30 minutes away.

25. Some responders want to wait until the airbags arrive, arguing that airbags are the best tool available for lifting tractors. Others want to lift the tractor with either the boom truck or hydraulic jacks. The ground beneath the tractor is firm. What is your opinion?

26. Describe the patient care you want to initiate prior to and during rescue efforts.

You and fellow responders are able to lift the tractor, free Mike's leg, and immobilize him to a long backboard. You note that he is extremely pale, and he now responds only to painful stimuli. You are unable to feel a radial pulse, so you take his carotid pulse, which is 140 beats per minute. His leg is badly crushed. An update from dispatch indicates that the helicopter has been delayed due to mechanical problems and may not be available for some time, if at all. The paramedic ambulance has responded from the nearest hospital and is still 30 minutes away.

27. Do you want to wait on scene or begin transporting the patient in the back of a pickup truck, rendezvousing with the ambulance or helicopter at some point? Explain your transport plan.

CHAPTER 22

INJURIES TO THE HEAD, FACE, AND NECK

KEY IDEAS

This chapter describes the assessment and emergency care of head-injured patients. It also describes injuries to the face and neck, which can compromise the patient's airway and signal severe facial or skull fractures and cervical-spine injuries. Key ideas include the following:

- One of the most important clues about the severity of the patient's head injury is the degree to which the patient's condition changes over time.

- If the mechanism of injury suggests a possible head injury, or if a trauma patient is unresponsive, suspect spine injury. Whenever you suspect head or spine injury, immediately stabilize the patient's head and neck. Maintain manual stabilization until the patient is completely immobilized.

- Injuries to the head include skull fracture, injuries to the brain, concussion, and penetrating wounds.

- Emergency care for head injuries includes supporting the patient's ABCs, stabilizing the patient's head and neck, and arranging for rapid transport to an appropriate hospital.

- Face and neck injuries can potentially compromise a patient's airway or breathing. Keep the airway the emergency care priority.

- It should be assumed that any patient with a significant face or neck injury also has a spine injury. Manually stabilize the patient's head and neck until he or she is completely immobilized.

- Do not attempt to remove foreign objects from ears or the nose. Never pack the ears or nose when attempting to control bleeding.

- Emergency care for injuries to the eye—including injuries to the eyelid or the bony structure around the eye—includes flushing out any foreign objects, controlling bleeding, and protecting the eyeballs from further injury.

CONTENT REVIEW

1. You are assessing a possible head-injured patient. His level of responsiveness, as well as pulses, movement, and sensation in his extremities, appear to be normal. List six special findings that could indicate this patient has suffered a head injury.

   a.

   b.

   c.

   d.

   e.

   f.

2. You have responded to a 34-year-old male who was struck in the head with a piece of lumber at a work site. He was briefly knocked unconscious. You and your partner find the patient awake but combative and vomiting. Your partner responds, "It's probably just a concussion. How bad could it be?" Do you agree with your partner's assessment? Explain.

3. Identify all the conditions listed below that should lead you to suspect spine injury:
   a. head injuries
   b. fever, nausea, vomiting
   c. significant facial injuries
   d. neck wounds

4. You should suspect spine injury in a medical patient who is unresponsive.

   _____ True

   _____ False

5. You are alone with a male patient who has significant head and lower-extremity injuries. How can you stabilize his head and neck and still provide emergency medical care for his wounds?

6. Why should you never apply direct pressure to a head wound that is accompanied by an obvious or depressed skull fracture?

7. Closed injuries of the head may present with which of the signs listed below? (There is more than one answer.)
   a. severe bleeding of the scalp
   b. clear fluid tinged pink from the nose
   c. leaking of cerebrospinal fluid from the ears
   d. swelling or depression of the bones of the skull

8. List three important details that should be included in a history of a patient with a head injury.

   a.

   b.

   c.

9. Change in a patient—not the patient's status at any one time—may be the most important sign of how a patient is doing.

   _____ True

   _____ False

10. The most frequent cause of death following a head injury is:
    a. loss of pulses in the extremities.
    b. oxygen deficiency in the brain.
    c. loss of cerebrospinal fluid.
    d. unresponsiveness.

11. Your priorities while caring for a patient with a head injury are included in the list below. Identify all of them.
    a. controlling major bleeding
    b. protecting the patient's cervical spine
    c. maintaining an open airway and adequate breathing
    d. arranging for rapid transport to the hospital

12. Suspect skull fracture with any significant trauma to the head, even if the injury is a closed one.

_____ True

_____ False

13. Which of the following factors most influences the severity of brain damage from a head injury?
    a. whether or not the skull is fractured
    b. the mechanism of injury and the force involved
    c. whether arteries rather than veins have been torn
    d. the length of time that elapses before the patient reaches the hospital

14. A _____ is a temporary loss of the brain's ability to function. Its key distinguishing feature is that its effects appear immediately or soon after impact.
    a. concussion
    b. skull fracture
    c. spine injury
    d. facial trauma

15. Your patient has been stabbed in the skull with an ice pick. It remains embedded. The wound is bleeding, but not profusely. How should you proceed?

16. After you have stabilized an object that is impaled in a patient's skull, you should permit blood to drain from the wound.

_____ True

_____ False

17. Which of the following are problems that can occur with severe facial injuries? (There is more than one answer.)
    a. blocked airway
    b. skull fracture
    c. spine injuries
    d. severe bleeding

18. Abrasions and lacerations to the face are soft-tissue injuries. They do not suggest underlying fractures.

_____ True

_____ False

19. List five signs and symptoms of injuries to the jaw.

a.

b.

c.

d.

e.

20. Management of a broken tooth includes which two of the following actions?
a. Wrap the tooth in a dry, sterile gauze pad.
b. Place the tooth in a cup of milk.
c. Clean the tooth with an antibacterial disinfectant.
d. Wrap the tooth in moistened gauze.

21. List five signs and symptoms of a neck injury:

a.

b.

c.

d.

e.

22. Is it appropriate to apply heavy direct pressure to control bleeding when treating a neck injury? Why or why not?

23. You are managing an unresponsive patient who received a severe laceration to her neck. She is having trouble breathing. Emergency care steps are listed below. Write 1–5 to show the correct order in which they should be performed.

_____ **a.** Apply a bulky dressing.

_____ **b.** Apply an occlusive dressing, and form an airtight seal.

_____ **c.** Apply 100% oxygen via nonrebreather mask. Be prepared to assist ventilation if needed.

_____ **d.** Open the patient's airway using the jaw-thrust maneuver.

_____ **e.** Manually stabilize the patient's head and neck.

24. Complete the eye assessment below by writing in the appropriate questions.

a. Eye orbits:

b. Eyelids:

c. Mucous membranes:

d. Globes:

e. Pupils:

f. Eye movement:

25. A patient has received a laceration to her left eyeball. Why should you cover both eyes with patches?

26. List two different methods for removing foreign objects from the eye.

a.

b.

27. You are managing a patient who has fragments of glass lodged in his eye. Describe the appropriate care for this injury.

28. If your patient has both an eye orbit and eyeball injury, place cold packs over the injured eye.

_____ True

_____ False

29. Which of the following eye injuries requires the most urgent and immediate care?
   a. scratched cornea
   b. fractured orbit
   c. chemical burn
   d. lacerated eyelid

30. Eyes contaminated with chemicals should be flushed with clean water for at least _____ minute(s) and _____ to _____ minutes are recommended.
   a. 1, 3, 5
   b. 3, 5, 10
   c. 10, 12, 15
   d. 20, 30, 60

31. A patient has a pencil impaled in her eye. This injury is best protected by:
   a. covering the eye and pencil with bulky dressings and roller gauze.
   b. cutting off the pencil and wrapping roller gauze around both eyes.
   c. placing a cup or cone over the pencil and securing it with roller gauze.
   d. leaving the injury alone.

32. Contact lenses should be removed when:
   a. there is a chemical burn to the eye.
   b. there is an injury to the face.
   c. the transport time is short.
   d. there is an impaled object in the eye.

Questions 33–35 refer to a 20-year-old woman, the driver of a car that plowed into a telephone pole. She was not wearing her seat belt and was thrown into the windshield. Her face and neck are badly torn up and bleeding. She has gurgling respirations.

33. You are met by one of the bystanders who extricated her from the car. "We've already called 9-1-1. We've got her on her back. She looks bad." What is your most immediate concern for this patient?
   a. managing her airway
   b. controlling bleeding
   c. protecting her spine
   d. treating her for shock

34. You have managed to clear the patient's airway and have positioned a bystander to manually support the patient's head and neck in a neutral position. Your next action would be to:
   a. place ice packs on the patient's face to reduce swelling.
   b. control the bleeding from her throat lacerations.
   c. apply cravat bandages to support her jaw fracture.
   d. complete a physical exam to check for other major injuries.

35. Given the mechanism of injury and your findings so far, what other injuries, besides those already listed, do you suspect?

CASE STUDY: BIKE RIDERS WITHOUT HELMETS

▼

Read the scenario and answer the questions that follow. Focus on the correct assessment of a head-injured patient and prioritize treatment, taking into consideration available resources.

There's "motorcycle down" on a narrow two-lane country highway. You arrive to find a "Harley Hog" wrapped around a telephone pole. Bystanders tell you that the bike, with two unhelmeted riders aboard, came around a sharp corner too quickly and slid into the telephone pole at high speed. The rider on the back of the motorcycle, a woman in her 30s, was thrown onto the blacktop. The driver, a male also in his 30s, stayed with the bike until it impacted the telephone pole. He was then launched into a guard rail.

As you gather equipment, you can see that neither patient is moving. As you approach the female patient, your partner, Marco, calls for additional resources and then attends to the male patient.

The female patient is lying on her back, moaning. Her eyes are open. "What's your name?" you ask as you kneel beside her. Her eyes flicker at the sound of your voice, but she continues only to moan. You see that she is covered with abrasions and has a large head wound above her left eyebrow. Her left lower arm and left lower leg are swollen and bent at unnatural angles. They appear to be fractured. She is pale but has a strong, rapid pulse. Her breath smells of beer. A bystander approaches you.

"Can I help? I've been trained as a First Responder," she says.

"Sure," you reply, "Grab a pair of gloves from the cab of our rescue unit and I'll put you to work."

36. Which of the following tasks would be most important for this bystander to accomplish?
   a. Gather splinting materials for the patient's fractures.
   b. Cover the patient's abrasions.
   c. Take the patient's blood pressure.
   d. Manually stabilize the patient's head and neck.

37. After you complete an initial assessment and treatment, your partner returns to your side. "The other rider is dead. He's pulseless and has brain matter showing. How bad is she?" he asks, motioning to your patient. You respond:
   a. "She has a change in mental status and several deformed limbs."
   b. "She appears to be moderately injured."
   c. "I'm not sure how bad she is. I need to get a set of vitals first."
   d. "Not too bad. She has a few broken bones and I think she's mainly drunk."

You perform a physical exam of the patient. She has bruising to her chest and abdomen. Her breathing is 26, pulse 120, blood pressure 116/88. You note that her breathing has a gurgling sound and discover that her mouth is filling with blood from a laceration inside the cheek. Marco has gone back to the rescue unit to grab a long backboard and bandaging supplies.

38. Your next action should be to:
   a. suction the patient's airway.
   b. apply high-flow oxygen via nonrebreather oxygen mask.
   c. reassess the patient's level of responsiveness.
   d. apply a cervical collar to the patient's neck.

39. After stabilizing her injuries, you move your patient onto the long backboard. At that time, you notice that her respirations have dropped to six to eight breaths per minute. These respirations are very irregular and shallow. Which of the following treatments would be appropriate for this patient? (There is more than one answer.)
   a. head-tilt/chin-lift and high-flow oxygen via nonrebreather mask
   b. mouth-to-mask ventilation with supplemental oxygen
   c. oropharyngeal airway and high-flow oxygen via BVM ventilation
   d. oropharyngeal airway and high-flow oxygen via nonrebreather mask

40. The paramedics have just arrived, and they are preparing to take over patient care. Give them a hand-off report on your patient. Make it brief.

41. As you assist the paramedics with strapping the patient to the backboard, you overhear them discussing whether or not they should fly the patient to the hospital by helicopter. A helicopter was dispatched when the paramedics were requested. At this point, helicopter transport would shave about 10 to 12 minutes off the transport time to the hospital. What do you think? How would you transport this patient?

CHAPTER 23

INJURIES TO THE SPINE

KEY IDEAS

This chapter focuses on spinal injuries. It covers the mechanisms of spine injuries, patient assessment, and emergency care. Key ideas include the following:

- Injuries to the spine can affect almost any body system. Improper handling of a spine-injured patient can kill the patient or cause permanent disability.

- Suspect spine injury in any patient with a head injury. If the mechanism of injury suggests a possible head injury, or if a trauma patient is unresponsive, suspect spine injury.

- If the mechanism of injury suggests it, assume a spine injury even if your assessment finds nothing wrong with the patient.

- Signs and symptoms of a spine injury can range from mild neck tenderness to paralysis and respiratory arrest.

- The goals of managing a spine-injured patient are to support the patient's ABCs and to stabilize his or her spine until the patient is completely immobilized.

▼

1. Complete the sentence below by filling in the missing words.

   The spinal cord is responsible for sending signals from the _____ to the

   _____ and receiving signals from the _____ and relaying

   them to the _____ .

2. The spinal column is made up of _____ bones, one stacked on top of the other.
   a. 11
   b. 22
   c. 33
   d. 44

3. The cervical spine is made up of 12 vertebrae and is supported by the rib cage.

   _____ True

   _____ False

4. The section of the spine most prone to injury is the:
   a. thoracic spine.
   b. cervical spine.
   c. lumbar spine.
   d. sacral spine.

5. Why should you suspect a spine injury in a patient with a head injury?

6. List four emergencies in which your index of suspicion for spine injury should be very high.

   a.

   b.

   c.

   d.

7. If the mechanism of injury suggests it, suspect spine injury even if there are no signs or symptoms.

   _____ True

   _____ False

8. The lack of back pain or the ability to walk, move arms and legs, or feel sensation rules out spine injury.

_____ True

_____ False

9. Your patient has a suspected spine injury. Immediately upon completing your _____ , stabilize her head and neck.
   a. scene size-up
   b. initial assessment
   c. physical examination
   d. ongoing assessment

10. List six signs and symptoms of a spinal injury.

   a.

   b.

   c.

   d.

   e.

   f.

11. For a physical exam of a suspected spine-injured patient's back, do NOT:
   a. palpate the patient's spine.
   b. bare the patient's chest and back.
   c. continue if upon palpation there is pain.
   d. ask the patient if his or her spine hurts.

12. A cervical-spine injury can result in severe breathing problems, even respiratory arrest.

_____ True

_____ False

13. Describe how you should assess pulses, movement, and sensation in all four extremities of a suspected spine-injured patient who is alert.

14. Describe how you can assess movement and sensation in a suspected spine-injured patient who is unresponsive.

15. Complete the paragraph below by filling in the missing words.

    To manually stabilize a patient's cervical spine, you must place your gloved hands just

    _____ the patient's ears. Then hold the patient's head

    _____ and _____ in a neutral, in-line position.

16. The word "neutral" in the term "neutral in-line position" means the head is:
    a. flexed forward and extended back.
    b. not flexed forward but extended back.
    c. flexed forward but not extended back.
    d. neither flexed forward nor extended back.

17. The word "in-line" in the term "neutral, in-line position" means the patient's:
    a. nose is in line with the chin.
    b. nose is in line with the navel.
    c. "Adam's apple" is in line with the navel.
    d. "Adam's apple" is in line with the chin.

18. If you find that the spine-injured patient's head is not in line, gently put it there, even if you feel resistance.

    _____ True

    _____ False

19. Manual stabilization must be maintained, even when the patient is immobilized from head to toe on a long backboard.

    _____ True

    _____ False

20. Even the best rigid cervical immobilization devices do NOT prevent movement.

    _____ True

    _____ False

21. You have arrived at the scene of a side-impact motor-vehicle collision. The patient is a male in his 30s who was the driver of the car that was hit. He is complaining of neck pain. Another First Responder arrived on scene before you and applied a cervical collar to the patient's neck. You note that the patient is sitting unattended on the curb, cervical collar in place. The other First Responder is getting an incident history from bystanders. What is your opinion of the care given to this patient? Does it adequately protect his possible neck injury? Why or why not?

22. You have responded to a "man down" call. You find an intoxicated patient, James, who gives you a conflicting story. He first states that he was assaulted, struck in the head with a tire iron, and thrown to the pavement. He then states that he was really just sleeping and that his assault story actually occurred a week ago. You see what may be relatively old lacerations and bruises on his head. You find that he is unsteady on his feet (from the alcohol?) and that his grip appears quite weak. During your exam, a buddy of his, Bob, walks up and tells you that James had indeed been sleeping, and that Bob called 9-1-1 because "James was breathing kind of funny." Bob also seems fairly intoxicated. Should you take spinal precautions or not? Explain your decision.

23. You are managing a patient who has suffered a possible neck injury when diving into a pool. You arrive at her side after she has been rescued from the water. She is conscious and complains of neck pain and tingling to her arms and legs. Read the following actions. Number them 1–14 to show the order in which they should be performed.

_____ **a.** Administer high-concentration oxygen to the patient.

_____ **b.** Apply a rigid cervical immobilization device.

_____ **c.** Identify the mechanism of injury.

_____ **d.** Immobilize the patient's legs.

_____ **e.** Immobilize the patient's torso.

_____ **f.** Immobilize the patient's head.

_____ **g.** Open the airway with a jaw-thrust maneuver.

_____ **h.** Pad the spaces between the patient and the board.

_____ **i.** Perform a log roll, and place a long backboard under the patient.

_____ **j.** Perform a physical exam, including assessment of pulses, movement, and sensation in all four extremities.

_____ **k.** Reassess pulses, movement, and sensation.

_____ **l.** Reassess pulses, movement, and sensation.

_____ **m.** Stabilize the patient's head and neck.

_____ **n.** Withdraw manual stabilization.

24. Which one or more of the following statements are NOT true?
   a. All patients with suspected spine injury must be immobilized on a short backboard.
   b. Rescuers may not move a spine-injured patient from the position in which he or she was found.
   c. Secure the patient's head first, torso next, legs last.
   d. While securing the patient to the backboard, maintain manual stabilization.

25. Manual stabilization may be released when a patient has been properly secured to a short backboard.

_____ True

_____ False

26. The procedure called "rapid extrication" may be performed in certain emergencies. Write three examples of such emergencies.

   a.

   b.

   c.

27. Removal of a helmet from a suspected spine-injured patient requires at least _____ rescuers.
   a. 2
   b. 3
   c. 4
   d. 5

CASE STUDY: DIVING ACCIDENT
▼

Read the case study and answer the questions that follow. Focus on protecting the patient's spine while completing other tasks necessary to manage the patient.

You are enjoying a peaceful day in the mountains when you suddenly hear screams for help coming from the direction of a nearby creek. You rush over to a small, deep pool that is popular with summer hikers and find a group of people crowded around a 16-year-old boy on a sand bar. He apparently dove into the pool and struck a small outcropping of rock with the top of his head. Fellow swimmers rescued him from the pool.

The patient, John, is lying on his back. Blood is seeping from a wound on the top of his head. One of his friends, obviously terrified, takes John by the shoulders and shakes him. "John, c'mon, get up buddy," he pleads.

"Don't touch him!" another of his friends screams. "Can't you see that he's hurt badly?"
You notice that two other ashen-faced friends are standing nearby.

28. Describe your approach to handling this situation. What might you do to get this scene under control?

29. What are your first top priorities in assessing and treating John?

You find that John is awake but confused. His airway is patent. He appears to be breathing adequately, but you see that his abdomen, not his chest, moves with each breath. His pulse is 88 and strong at the wrist. His only injury appears to be the head wound. Bleeding is controlled. John is able to move his left arm slightly, which is the only extremity movement you see.

30. As you are caring for John, an onlooker says, "It looks like he can move one of his arms. That's a good sign, isn't it?" Which of the following would be the best response to this question?
   a. "He may still have a permanent spine injury. It's too early to tell."
   b. "That sure is. Keep your fingers crossed that everything's going to be okay."
   c. "Spine injuries can get worse over time. We'll have to let the doctors sort it out."
   d. "Movement is good. Since we don't know the extent of injury, we're going to hold him very still until the paramedics arrive."

By now you have completed your initial assessment and physical exam, through which John's head and neck have been manually stabilized in a neutral in-line position. Rather than speaking in confused sentences, John has become unresponsive and his eyes gaze without focusing on anything. His pulse has dropped to 44 beats per minute, and his breathing appears more labored.

31. What can you do at this point to help John?

32. "He's getting worse!" one of his friends shouts. "Let's carry him up to the road so that he'll be closer to the paramedics when they arrive." Do you agree or disagree with this plan? Explain.

33. Paramedics have arrived. Give them a brief hand-off report about John, including information about the mechanism of injury, your assessment, and your treatment.

CHAPTER 24

MUSCULOSKELETAL INJURIES

KEY IDEAS
▼

This chapter focuses on assessment and emergency care of patients with injuries to muscles, joints, and bones. Key ideas include the following:

- Muscle, joint, and bone injuries are some of the most common injuries First Responders will encounter. They can range from minor ankle or knee sprains to life-threatening fractures of the neck or pelvis.

- Accurate assessment and aggressive treatment of musculoskeletal injuries can prevent permanent disability and death.

- Since it is not possible for a First Responder to distinguish between sprains and strains or dislocations and fractures, First Responders are to treat all musculoskeletal injuries the same way.

- Patients who have suffered critical injuries require the First Responder to arrange for rapid transport to the hospital.

CONTENT REVIEW

▼

1. List the four major functions of the musculoskeletal system.

    a.

    b.

    c.

    d.

2. The musculoskeletal system is made up of more than _____ bones and over _____ muscles.
    a. 200, 600
    b. 100, 300
    c. 50, 150
    d. 25, 75

3. Common mechanisms of musculoskeletal injury include what three types of forces?

    a.

    b.

    c.

4. With an indirect force, the energy of a blow:
    a. causes an injury at the point of impact.
    b. is sent in parallel paths away from the body.
    c. travels along a path away from the point of impact.
    d. turns one body part in a direction away from a connecting part.

5. An obvious injury, like a broken leg, may actually be one of several related injuries located elsewhere in the body.

    _____ True

    _____ False

6. List five signs and symptoms of musculoskeletal injury.

    a.

    b.

    c.

    d.

    e.

7. In an emergency involving musculoskeletal injury, you should stay focused on treating the patient's life threats. Once that is done, you can turn to limb-threatening injuries.

_____ True

_____ False

8. Explain the following statement: "Sprains, dislocations, and fractures are all treated the same in the field."

9. Your patient is lying on the side of a two-lane road after falling from her bicycle. There is an open injury to her left leg half way between the ankle and knee. What appears to be a broken bone protrudes from the wound. Number the following actions 1–8 to show the order in which they should be performed.

_____ a. Cover the open wound at the injury site.

_____ b. Assess for distal pulse, movement, and sensation.

_____ c. Complete a scene size-up.

_____ d. Splint the injured leg.

_____ e. Complete a physical examination.

_____ f. Reassess for distal pulse, movement, and sensation.

_____ g. Complete an initial assessment.

_____ h. Manually stabilize the injured leg.

10. Your patient has closed musculoskeletal injuries to the forearm. To check for a distal pulse, you must palpate the _____ pulse.
    a. radial
    b. tibial
    c. femoral
    d. brachial

11. Your patient has closed injuries to the ankle. To check for a distal pulse, you must palpate the posterior _____ or the dorsalis pedis pulse.
    a. radial
    b. tibial
    c. femoral
    d. brachial

12. The ability to move an extremity, such as wiggling fingers or toes, means that impulses from the _____ system can reach these points.
    a. nervous
    b. endocrine
    c. circulatory
    d. musculoskeletal

13. You must maintain manual stabilization of an injured limb until the patient is completely immobilized on a long backboard.

    _____ True

    _____ False

14. List five reasons for splinting a musculoskeletal injury.

    a.

    b.

    c.

    d.

    e.

15. A splint that completely surrounds the injured limb is a(n) _____ splint.
    a. rigid
    b. traction
    c. improvised
    d. circumferential

16. A splint made from any available material that can immobilize an injured limb is a(n) _____ splint.
   a. rigid
   b. traction
   c. improvised
   d. circumferential

17. The patient has an open angulated injury to the lower leg. The First Responder decides not to remove the patient's jeans before splinting in order to avoid moving the protruding bone and making the injury worse. Do you agree or disagree? If you disagree, write your reasons.

18. Complete the paragraph by filling in the missing words.

If a long bone is injured, immobilize it and the _____ above and below it. If

a joint is injured, immobilize it and the _____ above and below it.

19. List three problems that can be caused by improper splinting.

   a.

   b.

   c.

20. Which one of the following splints would NOT be appropriate for immobilizing a painful, swollen, deformed forearm?
   a. self-splint
   b. improvised splint
   c. circumferential splint
   d. pillow splint

21. You are managing a 14-year-old patient who has a closed injury to her forearm. The bone is bent at an angle between the elbow and the wrist. You attempt to straighten it by pulling gentle traction, but she screams, "Ow! It hurts!" What should you do?

22. You and your partner are managing a patient who has fallen and presents with an elbow injury. Your partner turns to you and states, "There's no way we can leave that elbow bent like that. We need to straighten it so that extrication will be easier." What do you think? Explain your answer.

23. Analyze the splinting strategies used to immobilize the following injuries. Decide if you agree or disagree. If you disagree, write the correct answer in the space provided.

   a. A broken humerus was splinted with a padded board that was secured with a roller bandage. A sling and swathe was used to support the arm.

   b. A broken forearm was immobilized by straightening the arm at the elbow and applying a cardboard splint that extended from below the wrist to just below the elbow.

   c. The fractured hand was splinted by flattening the palm side against a padded board splint and securing it with a roller bandage.

   d. The patient has an injured pelvis. He was secured to a long backboard with padding between his legs and a blanket on each side of his hips.

e. The fractured tibia was splinted by securing two padded splints on either side of the leg, one extending from the hip to below the foot and the foot was secured in place by a triangle bandage.

24. Body substance isolation (BSI) precautions are NOT necessary during a splinting procedure.

_____ True

_____ False

CASE STUDY: AUTO VS. BRIDGE ABUTMENT

▼

Read this scenario and answer the questions that follow. Focus on prioritizing the management of musculoskeletal injuries as well as on the correct technique for splinting.

You are on a Sunday drive in the country when you notice that a sedan has just crashed head-on into a concrete bridge abutment. After reporting the incident on your cellular telephone, you run over to assess the scene and the patients. The scene appears to be safe. The car has suffered severe front-end damage. The steering wheel is not bent. The windshield has been starred on the passenger side. There are three patients in the car. The status of each follows:

Patient A: 22-year-old male, driver of the car. Was restrained with a three-point seat belt. Complains of pain and swelling to his right ankle and lower left leg. Has a small bump to his forehead where he impacted the side window. Did not lose consciousness. Appears to have strong radial pulses. Skin signs appear normal. Has good distal pulses and sensation in all extremities.

Patient B: 21-year-old male, unrestrained front-seat passenger. Was hurtled against the windshield and dashboard. Presents as very combative, with a large bruise to his forehead. Has serious-looking chest injuries. Right humerus and forearm appear to be deformed. Severe pelvic pain with palpation. Has weak radial pulses. Skin is pale, cool, and moist.

Patient C: 23-year-old female, back-seat passenger. Was restrained with a three-point seat belt. Did not lose consciousness. Complains of pain and deformity to her left clavicle and wrist. Is also unable to straighten her left knee, which is swollen and painful. Has strong radial pulses. Skin is pale, warm, and dry. Has a good distal pulse and sensation in her arms. There are no pulses present at her left foot.

25. Order these patients from most (#1) to least (#3) severely injured. Explain how you arrived at your decisions.

    a. Patient A:

    b. Patient B:

    c. Patient C:

An EMT ambulance and two fire trucks arrive. A helicopter has also been dispatched. The patients are extricated and placed on long backboards. You move over to where rescuers are packaging Patient B for transport. You remember that his humerus appeared fractured during your exam, and you reach for splinting materials from an open first aid box. An EMT turns to you and says, "I appreciate your help, but that arm just gets strapped to his chest. Nothing more."

26. Why would this EMT say this? Agree? Disagree?

27. You assist with Patient C. You have already splinted her wrist and are trying to apply a sling and swathe to her injured clavicle. Every time you try to apply the sling and swathe, you move her arm slightly, causing her severe pain. "Just let me hold my left arm with my good arm," she suggests. Does this seem to be an acceptable alternative? Explain your answer.

28. Another rescuer attempts to straighten Patient C's left leg, but she screams when the responder tries to do so. Describe a splinting strategy for this injury.

29. Describe a simple technique for splinting Patient A's ankle injury.

CHAPTER 25

CHILDBIRTH

KEY IDEAS

This chapter describes the basic anatomy of pregnancy, the stages of childbirth, and assessment and management of both the baby and mother during and after delivery. Key ideas include the following:

- Childbirth is a natural, normal process. However, it is physically traumatic and complications to both the baby and mother do occur, though infrequently. While emergency deliveries do occur in the field, most mothers in labor are able to deliver their babies in the hospital.

- Childbirth is divided into three stages of labor: dilation, expulsion, and placental.

- First Responders must be able to determine whether or not birth is imminent.

- The role of the First Responder during delivery is to help coach the mother through the delivery and then to support the mother's and baby's airway, breathing, and circulation.

- First Responders may at some point manage a patient experiencing pregnancy or birth complications. Most pregnancy complications can lead to shock. Pregnancy complications most commonly involve a problem with the umbilical cord or the position of the baby prior to or during delivery. Other delivery complications may involve multiple or premature births.

CONTENT REVIEW

▼

1. Complete the crossword puzzle.

ACROSS

1. This cord may be tied or clamped after the baby is born.
3. The amniotic _____ is also called "bag of waters."
4. A premature infant may develop this condition if he or she loses any blood.
6. When the placenta is delivered, it is called the after _____ .
10. The organ that contains the developing fetus
11. A(n) _____ kit is a kit that holds obstetrical equipment.
12. There may be two of these in a multiple birth.
14. When the baby's head first appears, we say the baby is _____ .

DOWN

2. You may see _____ staining of the amniotic fluid.
4. The bloody _____ may be one of the first signs of labor.
5. The neck of the uterus
6. When a baby's buttocks or feet are born first, we call it a(n) _____ birth.
7. This condition may be called "poisoning of the blood."
8. A(n) _____ cord is one that appears before the baby does.
9. Bloody show is another name for the expulsion of the _____ plug.
13. The umbilical _____ is the unborn infant's lifeline.

2. The _____ is a disk-shaped organ on the inner lining of the uterus.
   a. vagina
   b. cervix
   c. placenta
   d. perineum

3. The _____ provides nourishment and oxygen to the fetus from the mother's blood. It also absorbs waste from the fetus into the mother's bloodstream.
   a. vagina
   b. cervix
   c. placenta
   d. perineum

4. A full-term pregnancy lasts approximately _____ days.
   a. 175
   b. 280
   c. 360
   d. 420

5. Complete the paragraph by writing in the words that are missing.

   After the egg is fertilized, it embeds itself in the lining of the _____ .

   Development of the _____ begins almost immediately. During pregnancy,

   the fetus receives nourishment through the _____ ,

   which is an extension of the _____ . Before delivery,

   the _____ usually breaks and discharges fluid. When the

   _____ is fully dilated, the baby is ready to be delivered. When the baby's

   head can be seen at the opening of the _____ , it is said the baby is

   _____ , which is a sign that birth is imminent.

6. Complete the sentence by filling in the missing words.

   During the _____ stage of labor, the placenta separates from the wall of the

   _____ and, usually, is then spontaneously expelled.

7. At the beginning of the dilation stage of labor, contractions commonly occur 10 to 20 minutes apart and last about _____ to _____ seconds each.
   a. 1, 2
   b. 5, 10
   c. 30, 60
   d. 90, 120

8. How do the contractions a woman experiences at the beginning of labor compare to the contractions when delivery is imminent?

9. Describe the technique for measuring the length and frequency of contractions.

10. If contractions are more than _____ minutes apart, the mother usually has time to be transported to a hospital.
    a. 5
    b. 4
    c. 3
    d. 2

11. If contractions are _____ minutes apart, the mother usually has no time to be transported to a hospital.
    a. 12
    b. 7
    c. 8
    d. 2

12. List five questions you might ask an expectant mother in order to determine whether delivery is imminent.

    a.

    b.

    c.

    d.

    e.

13. One way to tell if you should prepare for a normal delivery of the baby on scene is to examine the mother for:
    a. crowning.
    b. toxemia.
    c. rupture.
    d. dilation.

14. At what point will a woman in labor have an uncontrollable urge to push down?
    a. at any stage
    b. dilation stage
    c. expulsion stage
    d. placental stage

15. You are managing a patient who is in labor. She was sitting in a chair when you arrived. You have her get in a supine position on the floor, and she immediately becomes quite pale and lightheaded. What may have happened to this patient, and how can you remedy it?

16. Describe how you would provide a laboring mother with encouragement, support, and coaching. How could you make her feel more calm, reassured, and confident? Provide specific examples.

17. In which of the following positions should your patient be placed while in the first and second stages of labor?
    a. supine
    b. standing
    c. left lateral
    d. position of comfort

18. List the equipment that at a minimum should be included in your obstetrical kit.

    a.

    b.

    c.

    d.

    e.

    f.

    g.

    h.

    i.

    j.

19. To protect the baby and the mother from contamination and infection, all materials used during delivery should be sterile, or at least as clean as possible.

    _____ True

    _____ False

20. List five BSI precautions you should take prior to and after delivery.

    a.

    b.

    c.

    d.

    e.

21. Help the mother relax with each contraction. Since _____ causes muscles to tighten, have her _____ with each contraction.
    a. inhaling, exhale
    b. exhaling, exhale
    c. exhaling, inhale
    d. inhaling, inhale

22. During the expulsion stage of labor, have the mother hold her breath for _____ to _____ seconds when she bears down. Any longer will cause too much straining, broken blood vessels, and tearing of the area around the vagina.
    a. 1, 3
    b. 3, 6
    c. 7, 10
    d. 11, 15

23. To prevent an explosive delivery, you should:
    a. firmly press the mother's legs together.
    b. apply firm pressure to the vaginal opening.
    c. elevate the mother's buttocks 8 to 12 inches.
    d. apply very gentle pressure to the baby's head.

24. What should you do if the baby's head delivers and you see that the amniotic sac is still intact and covering the baby's face?
    a. Leave the sac alone. It will rupture at the appropriate time.
    b. Pinch the sac, and push it away from the infant's head and mouth.
    c. Immediately place your patient in a knee-chest position and transport her to the hospital.
    d. Cut the sac using a pair of sterile surgical scissors.

25. The infant emerges with the amniotic sac still intact. There is meconium staining. You break the sac and push it away from the baby's face. What should you do next?

26. Meconium staining is not a life-threatening event. Just be sure to suction out the baby's airway.

    _____ True

    _____ False

27. What should you do if after the baby's head delivers, you see that the umbilical cord is wrapped around its neck?
    a. Do nothing. The baby is in no danger.
    b. Immediately cut the cord to prevent strangulation.
    c. Use two fingers to slip the cord over the baby's shoulder.
    d. Apply pressure to the baby's head to prevent it from delivering.

28. The baby has delivered, but he is not breathing. What is the first thing you should do?
    a. Suction the mouth and then the nose.
    b. Provide artificial ventilation immediately.
    c. Hold the baby by the feet and slap his buttocks.
    d. Nothing. He will breathe on his own in a few minutes.

29. The baby is still not breathing. What is the second thing you should do?
    a. Provide tactile stimulation.
    b. Provide artificial ventilation.
    c. Provide both oral and aural stimulation.
    d. Nothing. He will breathe on his own in a few minutes.

30. The baby is still not breathing. What is the third thing you should do?
    a. Suction the mouth and then the nose.
    b. Provide artificial ventilation immediately.
    c. Hold the baby by the feet and slap his buttocks.
    d. Nothing. He will breathe on his own in a few minutes.

31. After the baby has been delivered, assist the mother with delivery of the placenta in the following way(s).
    a. Encourage the mother to bear down as the uterus contracts.
    b. Gently guide the placenta and attached membranes from the vagina.
    c. Gently tug on the umbilical cord to help the placenta pass.
    d. Massage the uterus to help it expel the placenta.

32. In a normal delivery, you can expect the mother to lose about _____ cc of blood.
    a. 500
    b. 1000
    c. 1500
    d. 2000

33. Your patient has delivered both the baby and the placenta and is experiencing heavy bleeding. Management strategies for this patient include all of the following EXCEPT:
    a. Pack the inside of the vagina with gauze pads.
    b. Place sanitary napkins over the opening of the vagina.
    c. Encourage the mother to begin breastfeeding, if she plans to do so.
    d. Massage the lower abdomen to help the uterus contract.

34. The primary goal(s) of managing both the mother and baby after delivery include:
    a. keeping them warm.
    b. regularly reassessing the status of their ABCs.
    c. keeping them in close contact to one another.
    d. assuring that they are both transported immediately to the hospital to be evaluated by a physician.

35. List three conditions that would require you to perform artificial ventilation on a newborn.

a.

b.

c.

36. The recommended time for assisting a newborn's ventilations is between _____ breaths per minute.
   a. 10–20
   b. 40–60
   c. 80–100
   d. 120–140

37. If the newborn's breathing and pulse are absent or if pulse rate is less than _____ beats per minute, then start CPR.
   a. 20
   b. 40
   c. 60
   d. 80

38. For CPR on a newborn, the rate of compressions is _____ per minute and the ratio of compressions to breaths is _____ .
   a. 120, 3:1
   b. 100, 5:1
   c. 100, 5:2
   d. 120, 3:2

39. What is the proper method for maintaining perfusion in the baby when a prolapsed cord occurs?
   a. Monitor the situation carefully.
   b. Immediately clamp and cut the umbilical cord.
   c. Gently push the head off the umbilical cord.
   d. Push the umbilical cord back into the vagina.

40. You are assisting with the delivery of a baby. Your partner is ready to apply gentle pressure against the baby's head as it delivers, when he shouts, "It's a breech birth! The baby's bottom is delivering first!" The buttocks and trunk deliver quickly, but the baby's head appears to be stuck in the vaginal canal. Your next course of action should be to:
   a. rush the mother and child to the hospital.
   b. very gently pull the at the baby's torso.
   c. form an airway for the baby with your fingers.
   d. slip your hand under the baby's head and pull.

41. When managing twin births, the primary reason why you must clamp and cut the cord is to:
    a. prevent bleeding to the second baby.
    b. move the first-born baby out of the way.
    c. prevent the twins from becoming entangled in it.
    d. avoid confusion about which cord belongs to which baby.

42. Which of the following is NOT true about premature babies?
    a. A premature baby is born before the 36th week of pregnancy.
    b. Premature babies are more susceptible to infection.
    c. They cannot tolerate losing even tiny amounts of blood.
    d. Premature babies should not receive supplemental oxygen.

CASE STUDY:
DELIVERY IN A STATION WAGON

▼

Read the case study and answer the questions that follow. Keep in mind that labor is a natural process, not an illness or an injury.

You are dispatched to a "delivery in progress" on a busy expressway and arrive to find a woman in labor in the back seat of a station wagon. Her frantic husband had attempted to drive her to the hospital—which is still about 10 minutes away—but stopped and called for help when it looked like she was going to deliver her baby in the back seat of the car.

Your patient is lying sideways on the back seat. She is calling out for her husband, who is nervously pacing by the front of the car. Sweat is pouring down her face, and in between contractions she moans softly.

43. What strategies would you use to gain control of the scene, your patient, and her husband?

44. You time her contractions and find that they are 6 minutes apart, lasting about 45 seconds each. The hospital is about 10 minutes away, and traffic is relatively light. The transporting ambulance is about 3 minutes away. This is your patient's first baby. Do you want to set up to deliver the baby or arrange for the ambulance to transport her to the hospital? Explain.

45. Ten minutes have passed. There is still no ambulance. Dispatch tells you that the ambulance has been caught in a heavy traffic snarl and will be delayed at least 10 more minutes. What patient exam or patient history information would help you to gauge how imminent delivery might be?

46. A gush of clear liquid splashes your patient's thighs. "Oh my God! What was that?" she screams. "Is the baby coming?" Explain to your patient what has happened.

47. Your patient now tells you, "I need to push. I can't help it. I've got to push now." You check her vagina and see that the baby's head is visible. Explain what is happening.

48. The ambulance has just arrived, and so has the baby. You note that the newborn is fairly blue and limp. She is not crying. You vigorously suction, dry, and stimulate the baby, but she still remains limp and unresponsive. What is the next step in resuscitating this baby?

49. Success! The baby is now crying. She has turned from blue to pink and appears to have good muscle tone. The exuberant father wants to close the doors of the station wagon and drive his wife and child to the hospital himself. After all, he says, she is already in the car. No sense in making a mess of the ambulance, too. Do you agree or disagree with his plan? Explain your answer.

CHAPTER 26

INFANTS AND CHILDREN

KEY IDEAS

This chapter identifies emotional needs of children and parents in pediatric emergencies, describes a pediatric physical assessment, compares pediatric and adult anatomy, and identifies treatment strategies for common pediatric emergencies. Key ideas include the following:

- When managing an emergency involving an infant or child, First Responders must deal compassionately with the adults who are affected by the child's illness or injury. The top priority, however, is the health and safety of the patient.

- Assessment of an infant or child patient is similar to adult assessment in many ways. However, First Responders must take into account differences in anatomy and developmental characteristics when assessing an infant or child.

- Pediatric patients compensate better for shock than adults do. They also tend to decompensate rapidly when their shock state becomes severe. Hypothermia will intensify the problems faced by a pediatric patient in shock.

- Respiratory distress is one of the most common pediatric emergencies. Treating the airway and breathing in an infant or child is the top priority in First Responder emergency care.

- Most cardiac arrests in infants and children are caused by airway obstructions or respiratory arrest. Effective resuscitation depends on diligent airway and breathing management and effective CPR.

CONTENT REVIEW

1. Complete the chart by writing in the missing information.

PATIENT	AGE RANGE IN YEARS
Infant	
Toddler	
Preschooler	
School Age	
Adolescent	
Adult	18 and over

2. The patient most likely to be quite fearful of separation from parents is the:
   a. infant.
   b. toddler.
   c. preschooler.
   d. school-age child.
   e. adolescent.

3. At this age, the _____ is very sensitive to peer pressure and may need to be reassured that what he or she tells you will be held in confidence.
   a. infant
   b. toddler
   c. preschooler
   d. school-age child
   e. adolescent

4. At this age, the _____ is very curious, so be especially alert to the possibility of poison ingestion.
   a. infant
   b. toddler
   c. preschooler
   d. school-age child
   e. adolescent

5. At this age, the _____ is likely to cooperate and be willing to follow the lead of parents and the EMS provider.
   a. infant
   b. toddler
   c. preschooler
   d. school-age child
   e. adolescent

6. At this age, the _____ may be scared and feel that what is happening is his or her fault.
   a. infant
   b. toddler
   c. preschooler
   d. school-age child
   e. adolescent

7. When a child is injured, the First Responder should view the situation as one that involves just the child, not the whole family.

_____ True

_____ False

8. Describe one technique that you might be able to use to respond to parents who are very upset.

9. You have been called to the scene of an injured 6-year-old girl. Her father refuses to let you help. You should:
   a. keep in mind that the parent may be correct.
   b. provide life-saving emergency care to the child.
   c. explain how the law looks upon a neglecting parent.
   d. distract him so your partner can provide care.

10. You arrive at the scene of a seizure. The patient, 18-month-old Katie, has been running a fever for the past 36 hours and reportedly had a generalized seizure lasting about 45 seconds. She is conscious and crying. Her mother is quite upset. Between sobs, the mother tells you that Katie has been undergoing some tests to determine whether she has a chronic seizure disorder.

Your partner, impatient with the mother's tears, cuts her off and states, "Ma'am, it looks like this is a simple seizure caused by a high fever. The paramedics are here and we need to get Katie moving to the hospital." Your partner then leads the mother to the front passenger seat of the ambulance "so that the paramedics can concentrate on taking care of Katie."

Critique his behavior. What would be an appropriate response to this parent's information and behavior?

11. Generally, as part of any scene size-up, you would ask "Why was EMS called?" and "What is the chief complaint?" What other scene size-up question should you be sure to ask the caregiver of a pediatric patient?

12. One way to assess an infant's or child's level of responsiveness is to see if the patient is oriented to time and place.

    _____ True

    _____ False

13. The single most important care you can provide for a pediatric patient is to ensure an open airway.

    _____ True

    _____ False

14. What are five signs of early respiratory distress in infants and children?

    a.

    b.

    c.

    d.

    e.

15. If an infant's respirations are less than _____ per minute or a child's are less than _____ , assist ventilations.
    a. 20, 10
    b. 40, 20
    c. 60, 40
    d. 80, 60

16. One way to assess circulation in infants and children is by palpating a pulse. Complete the sentences below by filling in the appropriate location of those pulse points.

    a. Palpate the infant's _____ pulse.

    b. Palpate the unresponsive child's _____ or _____ pulse.

    c. Palpate the responsive child's _____ or _____ pulse.

17. When a pediatric patient is not breathing and has no gag reflex, an _____ should be inserted to assist in maintaining an open airway.
a. a bulb syringe
b. oropharyngeal airway
c. nasopharyngeal airway
d. tonsil-tip suction catheter

18. List six SAMPLE history questions you would want answered by a sick infant's caregiver.

a.

b.

c.

d.

e.

f.

19. While caring for a five-year-old girl who has fallen feet-first about five feet onto ceramic tile, a First Responder asks the parents, "How does your daughter usually respond to pain?" Explain why the First Responder asked this question.

20. Pay attention to your overall impression of how the pediatric patient looks and acts. Your observations may tell you more about the status of patient than any vital sign.

_____ True

_____ False

21. Children sometimes breathe irregularly, so monitor respirations for _____ seconds to determine the rate.
a. 15
b. 30
c. 60
d. 75

22. Respiration rates in children alter easily due to emotional or physical conditions. So an increase over a previous rate is not significant.

_____ True

_____ False

23. Which of the following statements about pediatric vital signs is NOT true?
   a. Measure an infant's pulse at the brachial pulse point.
   b. If pulse is too rapid or too slow, assess for respiratory distress, shock, or head injury.
   c. Blood pressure is an early indicator of shock.
   d. If capillary refill takes more than two seconds, the child may be in shock.

24. For each of the following facts about pediatric anatomy, physiology, or development, list the implications for possible injuries, illness, or treatment. The first one has been completed as an example.

   a. Young children explore their world by putting objects in their mouth.

   Answer: Young children can experience foreign body airway obstruction. Always rule out foreign body aspiration with any young child complaining of difficulty breathing.

   b. Infants have proportionately larger tongues than older children and adults.

   c. Children have proportionately larger heads than adults.

d. Children have much less blood volume than adults.

e. A child's skin surface is large compared to body mass.

f. Children often have extremely short necks.

25. Your four-year-old patient's vital signs are respirations 36, pulse 146, and blood pressure 76/56. Are they within normal ranges?

26. List five signs and symptoms of shock in the pediatric patient:

a.

b.

c.

d.

e.

27. Always suspect a foreign body airway obstruction (FBAO) in any short-of-breath or unresponsive infant or child.

_____ True

_____ False

28. An asthma attack in an infant or child is a serious medical emergency. Describe First Responder emergency care.

29. What are the most common causes of cardiac arrest in children?
   a. elevated pulse rates
   b. shock or scarlet fever
   c. noisy breathing and hypothermia
   d. airway obstruction and respiratory arrest

30. List four signs and symptoms of circulatory failure in the pediatric patient:

a.

b.

c.

d.

31. You are alone, and your patient is an infant who is breathless and pulseless. Write the next two steps you should perform.

    a.

    b.

32. Your infant patient has just suffered a seizure. So you ask the parents if the baby has had seizures before. "Yes," the mother answers. What else should you ask immediately? List five questions.

    a.

    b.

    c.

    d.

    e.

33. Which two of the following actions would NOT be appropriate when managing a child who is actively seizing?
    a. Turn the child to one side to help clear the airway.
    b. Restrain the child to prevent injury.
    c. Administer oxygen holding a mask slightly away from the face.
    d. Suction the airway using a suction device.

34. All seizures in pediatric patients, even those associated with high fever, should be considered potentially life-threatening.

    _____ True

    _____ False

35. What do the letters SIDS stand for?

S:

I:

D:

S:

36. Which one of the following is NOT typical of a SIDS baby?
   a. between the ages of four weeks and seven months
   b. has had several recent illnesses
   c. was asleep when he or she died
   d. was born prematurely

37. SIDS is a preventable disease.

_____ True

_____ False

38. When on the scene of a possible SIDS baby, you should:
   a. try to find some concrete evidence of neglect or abuse.
   b. be careful to avoid suggesting that the parents are to blame.
   c. refuse to answer questions related to the infant's condition.
   d. avoid or keep to a minimum any interaction with the parents.

39. You find that your patient is an infant boy who is breathless, pulseless, stiff, and cold in his crib. You suspect SIDS. What questions do you need to ask? List six.

   a.

   b.

   c.

   d.

   e.

   f.

40. List five signs and symptoms of physical abuse in an infant or child.

a.

b.

c.

d.

e.

41. List five signs and symptoms of neglect.

a.

b.

c.

d.

e.

42. The First Responder arrives on scene to find a child with injuries that raise the possibility of child abuse. The First Responder says to the parent, "You need to know that I think you have abused your child, and I'm going to report you to the hospital staff and local law enforcement." Do you think this statement was appropriate? Why or why not?

43. To learn the reporting protocols for your EMS system in regard to child abuse and neglect, you must find out what six pieces of information?

a.

b.

c.

d.

e.

f.

44. Calls involving the injury or death of an infant or child have a way of affecting EMS rescuers very deeply. A CISD after the event can help. The letters CISD stand for:

C:

I:

S:

D:

CASE STUDY: SHORTNESS OF BREATH IN A KINDERGARTEN CLASS

Read this case study and answer the questions that follow. Remember that infants and children require different levels of explanation about what is happening to their bodies and what you are doing to help them. Remember that a simple, straightforward, reassuring approach is best!

You have been dispatched to a kindergarten class at the local elementary school for a five-year-old female who is having difficulty breathing. You arrive to find Lateesha sitting at her desk in a tripod position, eyes wide with fear, audibly wheezing. Her respirations are rapid and labored, her skin appears to be pale and grayish. Her teacher tells you that her pediatrician suspects that Lateesha may be developing asthma.

45. Lateesha's initial vital signs are as follows: respirations of 36, pulse of 146, BP of 120/86. Are these vital signs low, normal, or high for a five-year-old? If they are low or high, what would be normal?

46. List five questions you would like to ask Lateesha. Be sure to state them in a manner appropriate for a five-year-old.

a.

b.

c.

d.

e.

47. The paramedics have arrived, and you must give them a hand-off report. Write 1–8 to correctly order the information in your report to them.

_____ **a.** Lateesha is currently undergoing tests to determine if she has asthma.

_____ **b.** This is Lateesha. She is five years old. About 20 minutes ago, she became acutely short of breath.

_____ **c.** Lateesha's medical card states that she takes no medications and has no drug, food, or other types of allergies.

_____ **d.** We initially found Lateesha sitting in this chair in a tripod position, stating that she was having difficulty breathing, with labored respirations of 36, a pulse of 146, and a BP of 120/86.

_____ **e.** Lateesha was using some accessory muscles to breathe. She had audible wheezes and was able to talk in only two- or three-word sentences.

_____ **f.** We applied high-flow oxygen by nonrebreather mask. After a few minutes it appeared that Lateesha experienced some relief. However, she remains quite short of breath.

_____ **g.** Lateesha's mother has been called, and she should be here any minute.

_____ **h.** Lateesha said she became short of breath while playing chase on the playground.

CHAPTER 27

EMS OPERATIONS

KEY IDEAS

This chapter provides a brief overview of some of the operational aspects of out-of-hospital emergency care, including the six basic phases of an emergency response and emergency vehicle safety. Key ideas include the following:

- First Responders should have on hand equipment for airway and breathing management, bleeding control and bandaging, and patient assessment. Also, personal protective equipment is necessary.

- There are six general phases of an EMS response: preparation, dispatch, en route to the scene, arrival on scene, transfer of care, and post-run activities.

- Many First Responders spend a lot of time in traffic, both in cars and on foot at the emergency scene. A safety course and refresher courses are recommended.

- Driver safety depends in large part on common sense and good judgment.

- First Responders must never compromise their own safety.

- Once inside an ambulance compartment, First Responders must protect themselves. The techniques of hanging on and bracing allow for safer movement in the compartment. Securing the patient correctly can protect both the patient and rescuer.

CONTENT REVIEW

1. List three types of equipment you should have on hand for the management of a patient's airway and breathing.

   a.

   b.

   c.

2. List six types of equipment you should have on hand for the management of soft-tissue injuries.

   a.

   b.

   c.

   d.

   e.

   f.

3. Which phase is the formal beginning of an EMS response?
   a. dispatch
   b. preparation
   c. post-run duties
   d. arrival on scene
   e. transfer of care
   f. en route to the scene

4. During which phase will you first hear details about an emergency to which you are to respond?
   a. dispatch
   b. preparation
   c. post-run duties
   d. arrival on scene
   e. transfer of care
   f. en route to the scene

5. The emergency medical dispatcher may give specific, life-saving instructions to the caller to perform during which phase of an emergency response?
   a. dispatch
   b. preparation
   c. post-run duties
   d. arrival on scene
   e. transfer of care
   f. en route to the scene

6. List three items of information EMS dispatch will obtain from callers who report an emergency.

   a.

   b.

   c.

7. While you are en route to the scene of an emergency, you must do which three of the following?
   a. Know the exact location of the emergency.
   b. Report the number of patients and severity of injuries.
   c. Ignore the speed limits, stop signs, and yields.
   d. Notify dispatch when you begin your response.
   e. Wear seat belts at all times.

8. In which phase of an emergency response should you decide whether or not the scene is safe to enter?
   a. dispatch
   b. preparation
   c. post-run duties
   d. arrival on scene
   e. transfer of care
   f. en route to the scene

9. In which phase of an emergency response should you provide a patient hand-off report?
   a. dispatch
   b. preparation
   c. post-run duties
   d. arrival on scene
   e. transfer of care
   f. en route to the scene

10. List four basic ways you can improve driving safety on the way to an emergency scene.

    a.

    b.

    c.

    d.

11. When traveling at increased speeds, you should brake to a safe speed _____ the curve.
    a. before entering
    b. after entering
    c. after leaving
    d. before leaving

12. When traveling at increased speeds, you should stay _____ of a curve.
    a. on the outside
    b. on the inside
    c. in the middle
    d. in the fast lane

13. As you approach an emergency scene, disengage your seat belt so you can slip out of the vehicle quickly.

    _____ True

    _____ False

14. Whenever you respond to an emergency in a vehicle, use your headlights and your emergency lights even in the daytime.

    _____ True

    _____ False

15. If you have to alert oncoming traffic while parked, leave your _____ lights on.
    a. sirens
    b. emergency
    c. headlights
    d. tail lights

16. Once you turn off your lights and siren, you are no longer driving an "authorized" emergency vehicle and you are subject to the laws meant to govern regular traffic.

    _____ True

    _____ False

17. There are three precautions you can take to protect your hearing while riding in an emergency vehicle. List them.

    a.

    b.

    c.

18. Park alongside the crash scene to protect injured patients from oncoming traffic.

    _____ True

    _____ False

19. It is midnight and Anthony is at the scene of an emergency that involved falling debris. There are multiple patients, and at first glance some of them look critical. As Anthony enters the scene, he puts on his protective gloves and takes other necessary BSI precautions. He is already wearing his jump suit and heavy-duty work boots. What other protective gear, if any, should he be wearing?

20. You should have three goals when you channel traffic away from an emergency scene. List them.

a.

b.

c.

21. When riding in the patient compartment of an ambulance, you should never have more than _____ off a stable surface.
a. one hand or two feet
b. two hands or one foot
c. one hand or one foot
d. two hands or two feet

Questions 22–25 relate to the following scenario: As the first response Unit 957 arrives on scene, the First Responder is set to fling open the door and run to the patient, who is bleeding.

22. What should the First Responder do before opening the door?

23. How should the First Responder open the vehicle door?

24. Should additional responders exit through their ambulance rear door or side door? Why?

CASE STUDY: SCENE SAFETY

▼

Read the case study and answer the questions that follow. Focus on scene safety.

Rescue 723 is dispatched to a motor-vehicle collision. The dispatcher informs the rescuers that there are three patients in one vehicle who are believed to have critical injuries related to the head and chest. The scene is located at First and Division Streets in the village.

25. List at least five safety tips involved in the emergency vehicle response to the scene.

    a.

    b.

    c.

    d.

    e.

26. Once on scene, you note that police have not yet arrived to control traffic. If you were to perform that task, what would three of your goals be for rerouting traffic?

    a.

    b.

    c.

27. Describe how you would place cones or flares to redirect traffic.

CHAPTER 28

HAZARDOUS MATERIAL INCIDENTS AND EMERGENCIES

KEY IDEAS

This chapter focuses on how to recognize hazardous materials at the scene of an emergency and how to respond to this threat. Key ideas include the following:

- Hazardous materials are substances that pose a threat or unreasonable risk to health, life, or property if they are not properly controlled during manufacture, storage, transportation, use, or disposal.

- With 50 billion tons of hazardous material manufactured in the U.S. annually, hazardous material accidents caused by equipment failure, vehicle collisions, environmental conditions, or human error are inevitable.

- First Responder responsibilities in a hazmat emergency may include identifying the hazmat incident, establishing command and control zones, identifying the substance, and establishing a medical treatment sector.

- First Responders must never compromise their own safety when helping to manage a hazardous material incident.

CONTENT REVIEW

▼

1. Write the three types of dangers hazardous materials present:

   a.

   b.

   c.

2. Write three examples of hazmats commonly shipped in the U.S.:

   a.

   b.

   c.

3. Complete the sentence by writing the missing word(s).

   The U.S. _____ requires specific hazards labels to be put on packages and containers and hazard placards to be placed on the outside of vehicles.

4. Using the NFPA 704 system, a red placard with a "4" written on it would denote a:
   a. low-risk health hazard.
   b. high-risk reactivity hazard.
   c. high-risk fire hazard.
   d. moderate-risk fire hazard.

5. The letters MSDS stand for:

   M:

   S:

   D:

   S:

6. The NFPA 704 system was developed by the:
   a. National Fire Protection Association.
   b. Natural Fire and Prevention Agency.
   c. Nation's First Protection Agency.
   d. U.S. Department of Transportation.

7. The _____ is a toll-free 24-hour emergency phone service provided by chemical manufacturers.
   a. DOT placarding
   b. MSDS
   c. CHEMTREC
   d. NFPA 704 System

8. Which of the following information sources is NOT designed to help identify the contents and relative danger of a substance being carried on a truck?
   a. DOT placarding
   b. MSDS
   c. CHEMTREC
   d. NFPA 704 System

9. Which of the following resources provide helpful information for treating patients contaminated by hazardous materials? (There may be more than one answer.)
   a. MSDS
   b. North American Emergency Response Guidebook
   c. CHEMTREC
   d. regional poison control center

10. List the four levels of hazmat training for rescuers, and describe the level of training for each.

   a.

   b.

   c.

   d.

11. A First Responder's specific responsibilities at a hazmat incident are:

   a.

   b.

   c.

   d.

12. You are out shopping when you see a delivery truck carrying bottles of compressed gas crash into a parked car and overturn. A crowd of onlookers gathers close to the truck. You have no hazmat training. What actions should you take?

13. When arriving at the scene of a potential hazmat emergency, the first step is to:
   a. assess the situation from a safe command position.
   b. set up a triage area for potential victims.
   c. begin evacuation from the hot zone.
   d. call for additional resources depending on the nature of the hazmat emergency.

14. Write three possible visual clues to the presence of a hazardous material:

   a.

   b.

   c.

15. When you are called to a possible hazmat emergency, you should station yourself _____ and _____ of the scene.
   a. downhill, downwind
   b. uphill, downwind
   c. uphill, upwind
   d. downhill, upwind

16. Once you have stationed yourself, it is best to look at the possible hazmat scene through your:
   a. binoculars.
   b. closed window.
   c. face mask with HEPA filter.
   d. chemical-resistant jumpsuit.

17. When you report your position and the situation to dispatch, your report should include:

    a.

    b.

    c.

    d.

    e.

    f.

18. The area immediately outside the location of actual contamination is called the:
    a. hot zone.
    b. warm zone.
    c. cold zone.
    d. outer perimeter.

19. The location for all rescuers and equipment not immediately managing the hazmat emergency is known as the:
    a. hot zone.
    b. warm zone.
    c. cold zone.
    d. outer perimeter.

20. You and your partner have arrived at the scene of a hazardous materials incident. A tractor-trailer jack-knifed on the highway, spilling its liquid contents all over the roadway. After sizing up the scene from a distance, you are able to identify the substance as a strong acid. You can see that the driver is still sitting in the cab. He appears badly injured. Acid is bubbling forth from a large gash in the side of the tank. The hazmat team should be at the scene in 10 to 15 minutes. What actions do you wish to take prior to their arrival?

CASE STUDY: INCIDENT AT THE PACKING PLANT

Read this case study and answer the questions that follow. Always remember to ensure your own safety above all other considerations.

You have responded to a possible inhalation emergency at one of the local vegetable packing plants. The dispatch originally indicated that one patient may have been exposed. You arrive to find a chaotic scene. Workers are streaming out of one packing shed, while supervisors are running around, shouting instructions to each other. You find a group of about 20 workers just outside the shed, complaining of headache, dizziness, and some difficulty breathing.

"What's going on?" you ask one of the workers.

"I think there's bad air in this packing shed," she says.

"What kind of bad air?"

"Who knows? They use different types of gases at this plant."

"Was anyone contaminated by any type of liquid?"

"No, just something in the air."

21. Your first action at this point should be to:
    a. begin initial assessments of the workers.
    b. move the people away from the danger.
    c. go into the building to see if there are more patients.
    d. attempt to identify the gas causing the incident.

22. A supervisor tells you that he is pretty sure the gas in the packing shed is carbon monoxide. Based on this information, is it really necessary to establish hot, warm, and cold zones, or to have a hazmat team dispatched? Explain.

23. A packing plant supervisor tells you that the contaminated shed has been evacuated except for three workers who cannot be accounted for. Hazmat personnel are still five to seven minutes away from the incident. The supervisor and some of the workers want to reenter the shed to look for the missing workers. Do you let them in or do you deny access until the hazmat team arrives?

CHAPTER 29

MULTIPLE-CASUALTY INCIDENTS AND INCIDENT COMMAND

KEY IDEAS

This chapter provides an overview of ways in which EMS systems respond to multiple-casualty incidents and your role as a First Responder. Key ideas include the following:

- The key to managing emergencies with multiple patients is recognizing priorities and organizing your actions.

- The Incident Command System (ICS) provides a command structure through which to manage multiple-casualty incidents.

- The EMS sector functions in a multiple-casualty incident include triage, treatment, transportation, and staging.

- In a multiple-casualty incident First Responders size up the scene, establish command, request additional resources, and begin triage.

- Triage is a process of classifying sick and injured patients. It is used to determine the order in which each patient receives medical care and transport.

- Multiple-casualty incidents can have a severe psychological impact on both patients and rescuers. Strategies for managing these impacts increase the effectiveness of rescuers and help to lessen the long-term problems associated with critical incident stress.

CONTENT REVIEW

▼

1. A multiple-casualty incident is defined as any incident in which _____ or more patients are involved.
   a. 0
   b. 1
   c. 2
   d. 3

2. Describe the responsibilities of each of the following officers in an Incident Command System.

   a. Triage officer:

   b. Treatment officer:

   c. Transportation officer:

   d. Staging officer:

3. You are the first to arrive at the scene of a multiple-casualty incident. Your major goals are to:

   a.

   b.

   c.

   d.

4. You are the first EMS personnel to arrive at the scene of a high-speed, head-on vehicle collision involving two cars. Your first action should be to:
   a. begin initial triage.
   b. request additional resources.
   c. size up the scene and establish command.
   d. block off the roadway and set out flares.

5. During scene size-up of a multiple-casualty incident, to what seven questions must you find answers?

   a.

   b.

   c.

   d.

   e.

   f.

   g.

6. When resources arrive on the scene of a multiple-casualty incident and you are relieved by someone higher in the chain of command, you should report what five facts?

   a.

   b.

   c.

   d.

   e.

7. A common three-level triage system is called START. Write what the letters stand for.

   S:

   T:

   A:

   R:

   T:

8. In the START triage system, "Priority-1 Red" is given to a patient if he or she meets certain criteria. Identify those criteria from the list below.
   a. The patient is dead.
   b. Injuries are life-threatening.
   c. The patient is not seriously injured.
   d. The patient needs minimal care to survive.
   e. Risk of asphyxiation or shock is imminent or present.
   f. The patient can be stabilized without constant care.
   g. The patient can wait for treatment without getting worse.
   h. The patient has a very good chance of survival if treated and transported immediately.
   i. The patient has injuries that would be fatal even if he or she received treatment.

9. Use a typical three-level system to triage the following patients. Write "Priority 1," "Priority 2," "Priority 3," or "no care" after each one.

_____ a. A patient with shortness of breath and cyanosis

_____ b. A patient in respiratory arrest after repositioning the airway

_____ c. A patient with a painful, swollen ankle

_____ d. A patient in labor with an imminent birth

_____ e. A patient with an open, deformed injury to the right femur

_____ f. A patient with swelling and deformity to both arms

_____ g. A patient having a generalized seizure

_____ h. A patient who is unresponsive with no signs of head or spine injury

_____ i. A patient with superficial burns to a forearm

_____ j. A patient with uncontrolled bleeding from the wrist

_____ k. A patient with full-thickness burns on the hands

_____ l. A patient with generalized hypothermia

_____ m. A patient with a two-inch laceration to a calf with controlled bleeding

_____ n. A patient with hypoglycemia

_____ o. A patient with inhalation burns

_____ p. A patient with suspected ingested poisoning

_____ q. A patient with burns to the legs, pelvis, and chest

_____ r. A patient with cuts and bruises all over the body

_____ s. A patient with unknown trauma to both eyes

_____ t. A patient who is breathing but says it is very difficult

_____ u. A trauma patient with rapid pulse, cool moist skin that is gray looking, and altered mental status

_____ v. A patient with a closed wound to the head and altered mental status

_____ w. A patient who is unresponsive and pulseless

_____ x. A patient with broken ribs and a possible pneumothorax

_____ y. A patient with an abdominal evisceration

_____ z. A patient with severe blunt trauma to the cervical spine

10. As you begin triage using the START system, what is the first assessment you should conduct?
   a. If the patient is alert with no major bleeding, move on.
   b. Assess the patient's ABCs and treat them when they are found.
   c. Tell everyone to get up and walk unassisted to a specified area.
   d. If there is no carotid pulse, tag the patient as a "Priority-0 Black."

11. Using the START system, what is your initial assessment of the following patients? Write "Priority-1 Red," "Priority-2 Yellow," "Priority-3 Green," or "Priority-0 Black" below each one.

   a. The patient's breathing is faster than 30 breaths per minute.

   b. You clear the airway of a patient who is not breathing and breathing does NOT resume.

   c. You clear the airway of a patient who is not breathing and breathing resumes.

   d. Respirations are 28 and the carotid pulse is weak.

   e. Respirations and pulse are good, but the patient only responds to voice.

12. Describe common psychological reactions that rescuers experience after managing an MCI.

13. How can rescuers get help in dealing with the stress caused by managing an MCI after the incident is over?

14. List three strategies for reducing the stress rescue personnel experience during management of an MCI.

a.

b.

c.

CASE STUDY: HEAD-ON ON THE INTERSTATE

Read the case study and answer the questions that follow. Remember, establishing an organized approach that correctly sets priorities is the most important determinant of a successful MCI.

You respond along with two other First Responders in a rescue vehicle to a reported head-on collision on the nearby interstate. Your communications center advises you that the closest law enforcement and ambulance responses are approximately 15 and 20 minutes away, respectively.

You arrive on scene to find all lanes of the interstate blocked by the collision. It appears that a bread truck crossed the center median and collided head-on with a station wagon carrying six occupants. There is massive damage to both vehicles. Bystanders have set out flares. As the senior member of the rescue crew, you are the initial incident commander.

15. What initial information should you gather during your scene size-up? List a series of questions you would ask when gathering this information.

16. You have identified seven patients, six in the station wagon and one in the bread truck. Use a two-level system to triage them. Write "immediate" or "delayed" in the space provided.

_____ **a.** An unrestrained 18-month-old female who appears to be unresponsive after being thrown against windshield of station wagon. She presents with head and chest injuries, rapid breathing, and a faint brachial pulse.

_____ **b.** A 37-year-old male, driver of station wagon. Presents with an altered mental status, from repeating himself to being confused about what has happened. He is pinned by the steering column and has obvious chest injuries and leg fractures.

_____ **c.** A 38-year-old male, the restrained driver of bread truck. He presents as alert with significant facial lacerations and neck pain.

_____ **d.** A 34-year-old female, restrained front-seat passenger of the station wagon. She took the brunt of the bread truck's impact. She appears to be breathless and pulseless with massive head, chest, and pelvic trauma.

_____ **e.** A 14-year-old male, back-seat unrestrained passenger in the station wagon. He has painful, swollen, deformed injuries to both thighs. He also has closed abdominal injuries. He is responsive and screaming.

_____ **f.** A 9-year-old female, unrestrained back-seat passenger in the station wagon. She was ejected from the car on impact, and was found supine on the median with massive open head injuries and a grossly angulated neck. She is unresponsive and breathing three to four times per minute.

_____ **g.** A 12-year-old male, restrained back-seat passenger of the station wagon. He has severe abdominal and chest pain and painful, deformed forearms. He presents as alert and crying.

17. Which of the patients listed above would you consider to be your top-priority patient? Why?

18. Unfortunately, there is no helicopter service available. Bearing in mind that optimally one ambulance should transport only one critical patient, how many ambulances should you request for this incident? Why?

19. Fire, law enforcement, and ambulance resources begin to arrive on scene. You relinquish incident command and take over control of the EMS sector. You notice that since the change in command, confusion has broken out. Ambulance crews are making their way directly to patients without stopping at the staging area, firefighters are running into each other as they pull equipment, and law enforcement officers are yelling at passing motorists to stop rubbernecking. All you can think is, "This MCI just got worse." What can you do to solve this problem?

20. Order has been restored. You see that patients are being extricated, packaged, loaded, and transported efficiently. You notice one responder sitting on the tailboard of a fire engine with his head in his hands, quietly weeping. Describe how you would handle this situation and what resources you would use to help him.

CHAPTER 30

WATER EMERGENCIES

KEY IDEAS

This chapter provides an overview of water rescue and water-related emergencies, including water hazards and how to provide emergency care in water. Key ideas include the following:

- Drowning is the third leading cause of accidental death in the U.S. After auto collisions, it is the most common cause of preventable death among children.

- The top priority in managing patients with water emergencies is the safety of the rescuer. The next priority is resuscitating the patient as soon as possible.

- Never attempt a water rescue unless you are a good swimmer, you are specially trained in water rescue, you are wearing a personal flotation device, and you are accompanied by other rescuers.

- Always assume that unresponsive patients have spine injuries. Patients with suspected spine injuries should have their spines stabilized while still in the water if possible.

- Barotrauma occurs when divers experience increasing underwater pressures or when they ascend from deep water improperly. Common types of barotrauma include air embolism, decompression sickness, and a phenomenon known as "the squeeze." Care for these emergencies focuses on supporting the patient's ABCs and transporting the patient to an appropriate hospital. Air-embolism or decompression-sickness patients should be transported to a facility with a decompression chamber.

1. There is a significant difference between warm- and cold-water drownings. Describe what that difference is in the space below.

2. Do not walk in fast-moving water over _____ depth, because it is not safe. Moving water can push you over and hold you down.
   a. knee
   b. waist
   c. mid-chest
   d. shoulder

3. Which of the following items pose a hazard for water rescuers? (There is more than one answer.)
   a. oil or gas
   b. blood
   c. sewage
   d. electricity

4. Questions you should ask during size up of a water emergency include those related to the condition of the water. Identify all such questions from the list below.
   a. Are there hazardous materials or conditions present?
   b. Can you see any potential hazards under the water?
   c. Can your feet touch the bottom so you can stand?
   d. How many rescuers are trained and on scene?
   e. Is the patient on the surface or is he submerged?
   f. Is the patient responsive and able to assist in rescue?
   g. Will the location of the patient change?

5. Never try a water rescue unless you meet all of four basic criteria. List them.

   a.

   b.

   c.

   d.

6. You are enjoying a sunny afternoon at a lake when you hear that a swimmer is in trouble just offshore. You run over to where a group of people have gathered. You see a woman in her 20s thrashing about in the water about 25 yards offshore. Witnesses tell you that she was floating on an inflatable raft that lost air and sank. List three techniques that can be used to rescue her.

a.

b.

c.

7. You are working as a First Responder for an ocean rescue team and respond to a swimmer in distress. You arrive with two other rescuers in a motorized dingy. The ocean water is calm but quite cold. You find the patient face down 50 yards from shore, unconscious, breathless, and with a slow pulse. Number the following actions 1–8 to correctly order the steps for managing this patient.

_____ a. Continue artificial ventilation.

_____ b. Turn the patient onto his back, keeping his neck and back aligned.

_____ c. Float a board beneath the patient, secure the patient to it, and load the patient onto the boat.

_____ d. Initiate rescue breathing.

_____ e. While you are waiting for an ambulance, perform a physical exam and gather a patient history.

_____ f. Suction the patient using a suction device.

_____ g. Perform an initial assessment.

_____ h. Reassess the patient's ABCs.

8. Your patient is unresponsive and face down in shallow water. To turn him, you should use the _____ technique.
   a. head-splint
   b. recompression
   c. reach-and-throw
   d. head-chin support

9. To turn a patient face up in deep water, you should use the _____ technique.
   a. head-splint
   b. recompression
   c. reach-and-throw
   d. head-chin support

10. You are rescuing a responsive near-drowning patient who is in safe, shallow water. Your first action should be to:
    a. perform a physical exam.
    b. activate the EMS system.
    c. perform an initial assessment.
    d. administer high-flow oxygen.
    e. remove the patient from the water.
    f. conserve the patient's body heat.

11. A drowning patient is unresponsive, breathless, and pulseless and in water that is shallow, but cold and moving fast. Decide whether the following statements are true or false:

    a. Only qualified rescuers—that is, rescuers, who are properly equipped and trained—may enter the water for a rescue.

       _____ True

       _____ False

    b. Because of the patient's critical condition, rescuers may remove him from the water without stabilizing his head and spine.

       _____ True

       _____ False

    c. Rescuers must start CPR on this patient immediately, but not until the patient is removed from the water.

       _____ True

       _____ False

    d. When the patient's spine is immobilized on a long backboard, the rescuers should leave the patient's lifejacket in place.

       _____ True

       _____ False

12. Near-drowning patients should always be transported to the hospital because:
    a. you may miss an important finding during your assessment.
    b. they require sophisticated tests to make sure they are okay.
    c. they always need hospitalization regardless of their status.
    d. complications can develop up to 72 hours after the incident.

13. Which of the following would NOT be appropriate care for a neck-injured, near-drowning patient still in the water?
    a. Ventilate the patient only after removing her from the water.
    b. Keep her floating on her back until further help arrives.
    c. Support her head and neck level with her back.
    d. Do not remove the patient from the water until help arrives.

14. The force of moving water can be measured solely by its velocity.

    _____ True

    _____ False

15. Fast-moving water is dangerous. Certain river features make it even more so. Write a brief description of the dangers each one listed below may pose.

    a. Strainers:

    b. Obstructions:

    c. Recirculating currents or "holes":

    d. Low-head dams:

16. A swimmer fell into fast water and experienced a foot entrapment. What can you tell him is the best thing to do until he is rescued?
    a. Do a back stroke with feet pointed downstream.
    b. Pull out your foot in any way except the way it went in.
    c. Dive down and try to pull out your foot with your hands.
    d. Breathe through a straw that reaches the water's surface.

17. A good rule to follow for an ice rescue is: "one inch, keep off; two inches, one may; three inches, small groups; four inches, okay."

_____ True

_____ False

18. Describe how the following water-rescue techniques apply to ice rescue.

    a. Reach and Throw:

    b. Row:

    c. Go:

19. Air embolism usually occurs when:
    a. a diver holds his or her breath during a dive.
    b. a diver comes up too quickly from a deep, prolonged dive.
    c. air pressure is not equalized in the body's air cavities.
    d. a diver stays submerged for too long.

20. Which one of the following is the correct position in which to place an uninjured patient with signs of air embolism?
    a. supine
    b. sitting up, with legs in a dependent position
    c. left lateral, with head and chest lower than feet
    d. prone

21. Decompression sickness usually occurs when:
    a. a diver holds his or her breath during a dive.
    b. a diver comes up too quickly from a deep, prolonged dive.
    c. air pressure is not equalized in a body's air cavities during ascent or descent.
    d. a diver stays submerged for too long a period of time.

22. Which of the following statements regarding decompression sickness is NOT true?
    a. When the diver ascends, nitrogen turns into tiny bubbles that lodge in the body's tissues.
    b. Nitrogen bubbles eventually enter the bloodstream and can cause injuries to major organs.
    c. The risk of decompression sickness increases if the diver flies in an airplane shortly after diving.
    d. The signs and symptoms of decompression sickness occur rapidly following the dive.

23. "The squeeze" usually occurs when:
   a. a diver holds his or her breath during a dive.
   b. a diver comes up too quickly from a deep, prolonged dive.
   c. air pressure is not equalized in a body's air cavities during ascent or descent.
   d. a diver stays submerged for too long a period of time.

CASE STUDY: "CHILD IN THE WATER, POSSIBLE DROWNING"

Read the scenario and answer the questions that follow. Remember that effective resuscitation of a patient depends on an accurate assessment and aggressive treatment of the patient's airway, breathing, and circulation.

You have just finished lunch at the fire station when one of the calls you dread the most is dispatched: "Child in the water, possible drowning." As you respond to a nearby resort, your dispatcher updates you, stating that lifeguards have located an unresponsive five-year-old in the lake. A paramedic ambulance is approximately 10 minutes behind you.

24. What sort of management planning could you complete with your two fellow crew members en route to this call? How might you divide the workload for this call among the three of you?

As you drive up to the scene, two of the resort lifeguards are just exiting the water, carrying the child. One of the lifeguards is performing rescue breathing. A crowd of about 10 people converges on them, and they are lost from sight.

25. What actions should you take to get control of this scene?

You have controlled the crowd and have gained access to the patient. She is unresponsive, breathless, pale, and cold to the touch. The exhausted lifeguards continue to perform artificial ventilation. You ready your airway and ventilation equipment. "Does she have a pulse?" you ask.

"I think so," says one of the guards. You note that a pulse has not been checked on the girl since the lifeguards reached the beach. You also note that the lifeguard's ventilations do not appear to be achieving any chest rise.

26. What actions do you want to take at this point? Explain them in their proper sequence.

Your patient has a radial pulse of 50. You have cleared her airway and have taken over rescue breathing via bag-valve-mask supplied with 100% oxygen. You decided to use a jaw-thrust maneuver to open her airway, and you inserted an oropharyngeal airway.

Despite several attempts, you are not able to achieve adequate ventilations. Your patient has minimal chest rise with ventilation. You are somewhat concerned that she may have some sort of spinal injury, but you find yourself becoming more concerned with the lack of chest rise with ventilations.

27. List three methods you would use to open her airway and achieve adequate ventilations.

    a.

    b.

    c.

28. One of her parents approaches you and asks, "How is Maggie doing? Is she going to be all right?" At this point, Maggie's heart rate is 50 beats per minute. She is unresponsive and still breathless. The paramedics are about one minute away. Write out a short response to this parent.

29. The paramedics have just shown up. Number the following sentences 1–7 in order to develop a coherent, efficient report.

_____ **a.** Maggie remains unresponsive. She is not breathing on her own, but does have a strong radial pulse of 88.

_____ **b.** When we arrived, Maggie was unresponsive, with a slow radial pulse.

_____ **c.** Maggie is an unresponsive, near-drowning victim. She was submerged for about three to four minutes.

_____ **d.** The lifeguards spotted her about 20 feet offshore in about three feet of water. They rescued her and began rescue breathing immediately.

_____ **e.** We suctioned her airway, inserted an oropharyngeal airway, and began ventilating with 100% oxygen via BVM.

_____ **f.** We do not find any associated trauma.

_____ **g.** Maggie has no medical history, takes no medications, and has no medication allergies.

CHAPTER 31

VEHICLE STABILIZATION AND PATIENT EXTRICATION

KEY IDEAS

▼

This chapter provides an overview of vehicle stabilization and patient extrication and how you can proceed safely and effectively. Key ideas include the following:

- Safety is always the top priority when extricating a patient. Never attempt extrication or stabilization procedures that you have not been specifically trained to do.

- All EMS responders working in and around a wrecked vehicle should wear the proper personal protective equipment.

- The most important initial action when faced with an extrication problem is to size up the scene, determining the number of patients, the presence of any scene hazards, and whether or not you have the proper resources for managing the extrication.

- Suspect any vehicle of being unstable until you make it stable.

- Doors and windows provide simple access to patients. If complex access is required, call for rescuers who have the training and equipment.

- Spinal precautions should be taken on all patients prior to extrication.

1. You have responded to a vehicle collision. You drive up to find that a pickup truck has slammed into a telephone pole. The single occupant, a male in his 30s, appears awake but dazed. The windshield of the truck is starred, and the steering column is bent. There appears to be no fire danger. You radio in for a fire and ambulance response. What steps should you take to manage the scene and the patient prior to the arrival of these other resources?

2. What type of clothing should you wear when assisting with a vehicle extrication?

3. List five techniques for determining the number of patients at the scene of a vehicle collision.

   a.

   b.

   c.

   d.

   e.

4. Two goals of traffic control at the scene of a vehicle wreck are to:
   a. stop all traffic in order to maintain scene safety.
   b. reduce the flow of traffic by routing vehicles back the way they came.
   c. clear the scene of unnecessary vehicles so that emergency vehicles can gain access quickly.
   d. route traffic around the scene in order to prevent traffic snarls and secondary collisions.

5. Flares should be arranged by keeping in mind which of the following guidelines? (There may be more than one answer.)
   a. Flares should lead vehicles around the scene and help to keep traffic moving.
   b. The danger zone around the emergency site extends to a 50-foot radius around the wrecked cars.
   c. If the crash occurred below a hill, the danger zone should extend to the crest of the hill.
   d. If the crash occurred on a curve, the danger zone should extend to the start of the curve.

6. Flares should be set _____ feet apart.
   a. 3–5
   b. 10–15
   c. 30–45
   d. 100

7. Flares should extend _____ feet toward traffic.
   a. 10
   b. 25
   c. 50
   d. 75

8. Assume a vehicle at a crash site is NOT stable if what five conditions exist?

   a.

   b.

   c.

   d.

   e.

9. Which one of the following statements about cribbing is NOT correct?
   a. Cribbing is used to prop up vehicles.
   b. There should be no more than one or two inches between the cribbing and the vehicle.
   c. Vehicles may be cribbed under the wheels or tires.
   d. Wood is stacked in boxlike squares and wedges to keep pressure under the vehicle uniform.

10. Identify the steps you should take to stabilize an upright vehicle that rests on all four wheels.
    a. Place the gear shift in park.
    b. Chock wheels tightly against the curb.
    c. Crib under the frame, wheels, and tires.
    d. Cut the tire valve stems so the car rests on the rims.
    e. Place a solid object between the roof and the roadway.
    f. Use a bumper jack to angle it against a solid object.
    g. Use blocks at wheels to prevent unexpected rolling.

11. Complex access is access by which no tools are needed. Simple access is access that requires tools and specialized equipment.

_____ True

_____ False

12. An EMS responder is on the scene of an "auto vs. tree" and finds the vehicle with massive front and side damage. The patient inside appears to be unconscious with labored respirations. The EMS responder realizes that this patient needs airway and breathing management immediately. Provided the vehicle is properly stabilized, the two best methods for accessing this patient would be:
    a. attempting entry through a door.
    b. breaking a side or rear window.
    c. removing the windshield.
    d. cutting through the top of the car.

13. In order to gain access to your patient, you must remove one of the crash car's side windows. Number the following steps 1–7 in the order in which you should proceed.

    _____ a. Cover the patient with a blanket, if possible.

    _____ b. Draw the knife across the top and down the side.

    _____ c. Insert the point of a linoleum knife into the molding at the midpoint of the glass.

    _____ d. Pivot the window on its bottom edge.

    _____ e. Loosen the short pry bar behind the glass.

    _____ f. Remove the glass.

    _____ g. Repeat on the other side.

14. If you must break a window to gain access to a patient trapped in a crashed vehicle, break the window farthest from your patient.

    _____ True

    _____ False

15. Correct management of a car's air bag includes which two actions listed below?
    a. cutting the yellow air bag connector
    b. cutting the negative wires for the car's battery
    c. disconnecting the negative side of the car's battery
    d. disconnecting the yellow air bag connector

16. Which one of the following shows the correct order for extricating a patient in a sitting position from a stable car?
    a. stabilize head and neck, apply cervical collar, apply short board, place on long board, extricate.
    b. stabilize head and neck, apply cervical collar, apply short board, extricate.
    c. stabilize the head and neck, apply cervical collar, apply long board, extricate.
    d. stabilize the head and neck, apply short board, apply cervical collar, extricate.

17. You are at the scene of a "car vs. telephone pole." Your patient, the driver, is alert but cannot extricate his feet from beneath the dash. What strategy might you try first to help to extricate this patient?

CASE STUDY: MULTIPLE-PATIENT EXTRICATION

▼

Read the case study and answer the questions that follow. Remember that when faced with multiple-patient extrications, rescuers must prioritize the patients by the degree of injury as well as by the order of extrication.

You respond to a single-vehicle crash in which a sedan has collided with a bridge abutment. You arrive along with two rescuers to find a sedan with massive front and right-side damage. The sedan has come to rest with its right side wedged against the abutment. There are five occupants, two in the front and three in the back.

While one of your partners sets out flares, you size up the scene. The car appears to be stable. Radiator fluid is leaking, but there does not appear to be any fuel leakage or fire danger. The left side doors of the sedan will not open. You are unable to access the right side of the car. The windows of the car have been broken. You see that the front-seat occupants are trapped by the dashboard and steering column. They appear to have critical injuries. The back-seat occupants have fared better. They have moderate to severe injuries.

You update EMS dispatch, calling for additional ambulances and the heavy rescue unit.

18. Use a two-level triage system to prioritize your patients. Write "immediate" or "delayed" after each one. Then order them 1–5 to indicate the sequence in which you wish to manage these patients.

_____ a. **Chris:** 25-year-old restrained male, driver, trapped by steering column and dashboard; appears unconscious with gurgling, snoring respirations; has major head and chest injuries.

Priority: _____

_____ b. **Jim:** front-seat passenger, 23-year-old restrained male, also trapped by the dashboard; appears to be alert, with major abdomen, pelvic, and leg injuries.

Priority: _____

_____ c. **Sherri:** back-seat driver's-side passenger, 22-year-old restrained female; conscious with lacerations, bumps, and bruises, neck and back pain.

Priority: _____

_____ d. **Michael:** back-seat middle passenger, 27-year-old restrained male; conscious with large bump to the head, neck pain, and a swollen, deformed left forearm.

Priority: _____

_____ e. **Holly:** back-seat passenger's side, 26-year-old restrained female; major facial lacerations, swollen and deformed jaw, swollen, deformed right collarbone, neck pain.

Priority: _____

19. No additional emergency services personnel are on scene yet. One of your crew is still setting out flares and diverting traffic around the scene. You and your remaining crew member have pulled out your medical equipment. What assessment and treatment tasks should the two of you attempt to accomplish?

Additional personnel have arrived. Law enforcement takes over traffic control. You have a newly arrived First Responder set up a staging and treatment area for the incoming rescue units and ambulances. The captain of the heavy rescue unit tells you that it will require heavy rescue tools to extricate your patients. He tells you that he can have the left rear door of the sedan opened in about five minutes, but that it will take 20 to 30 minutes to pull the steering wheel and dashboard off the front-seat occupants.

20. Given this information, describe the order in which you wish to extricate the patients.

21. While the front-seat patients are being extricated, what type of assessment and treatment do you want to perform on them?

22. The rescue crew frees Chris from behind the steering wheel of the car. Describe how you would extricate him and what type of equipment you would use.

CHAPTER 32

SPECIAL RESCUE SITUATIONS

KEY IDEAS

This chapter provides an introduction to special rescue situations and hazards. Key ideas include the following:

- Lack of understanding about scene hazards can result in injury or death.

- Confined spaces pose hazards such as engulfment, suffocation, poisoning, electrocution, and drowning.

- In a trench collapse, a special team is necessary for the rescue. Note that one trench collapse carries a high potential for a secondary collapse.

- Prepare for a litter carry. A total of 18–20 rescuers are necessary to properly effect a carry over one mile. This allows teams to rotate positions and rest.

- Rough terrain increases the risk that a patient will be dropped or a rescuer injured. Identify low-angle or high-angle rescue situations and call for appropriate personnel.

- Helicopters can be called for either operational reasons or medical reasons. In both cases, the patient's condition indicates a need for rapid transport or transport to a specialized facility.

CONTENT REVIEW

▼

1. Define the term "confined space."

2. List three examples of confined spaces.

   a.

   b.

   c.

3. As a First Responder, your responsibility in a confined-space emergency is to quickly:
   a. recognize it and call for specialized help.
   b. provide life-saving emergency care to the patient.
   c. make sure the responders on scene are wearing SCBAs.
   d. lock and lag out all related electrical systems.

4. The tasks you should perform during a size-up of an enclosed-space emergency are listed below. Identify the task you should NOT perform.
   a. Call for a specialized rescue team.
   b. Determine what the hazards are.
   c. Establish safety zones.
   d. Obtain a copy of the permit for the site.
   e. Perform an emergency move of the patient.
   f. Determine how many workers are involved.

5. To avoid unnecessary emergencies, OSHA requires a "trench box" or "shoring" in any trench that is deeper than _____ feet.
   a. 3
   b. 5
   c. 7
   d. 9

6. In a cave-in emergency, the weight of two feet of soil on the patient's chest can equal about _____ pounds.
   a. 10,000
   b. 1000
   c. 100
   d. 10

7. No matter how a cave-in occurs, if the trench is more than _____ deep, a specialized trench rescue team is required.
   a. ankle
   b. knee
   c. waist
   d. chest

8. In a rough-terrain evacuation, it takes about _____ people to carry a patient on a portable stretcher for one mile.
   a. 18–20
   b. 14–16
   c. 10–12
   d. 6–8

9. Identify two items listed below that do NOT describe a high-angle rescue.
   a. The rescuers' hands are needed for balance.
   b. The slope forms more than a 40-degree angle.
   c. Rappelling is required to get down the slope.
   d. A fall would likely result in serious injury or death.
   e. The slope forms less than a 40-degree angle.

10. List three operational reasons for calling for a helicopter to the emergency scene.

    a.

    b.

    c.

11. Among the medical reasons for calling for a helicopter evacuation is a serious mechanism of injury. Write five examples.

    a.

    b.

    c.

    d.

    e.

12. A helicopter landing zone should be at least _____ feet.
    a. 25 by 25
    b. 50 by 50
    c. 75 by 75
    d. 100 by 100

13. In addition to being flat, a helicopter landing zone must have four more characteristics. List them.

    a.

    b.

    c.

    d.

14. Describe the correct procedure for approaching a helicopter.

The next two questions refer to Andrew, who has been injured while hiking in the mountains. He is currently lying on a ledge with a slope of 60 degrees. The ledge is approximately one mile from the closest road.

15. Will any special teams be needed to remove Andrew from the ledge? If so, which ones? Explain your answer.

16. Describe how you will plan to remove Andrew by stretcher to the roadway for transport.

CASE STUDY:
"TRUCK VS. TREE"

Read this case study and answer the questions that follow. Always remember to ensure your own safety above all other considerations.

You have arrived at the scene of a "truck vs. tree" on a very rural stretch of Route 202. As you approach the scene on foot, you see a tree broken off approximately four feet up from the ground and leaning precariously. There appears to be a female driver of the vehicle, and the vehicle has sustained extensive front-end damage. Even from a distance, you can see that the steering wheel is bent down toward the driver's chest. You can hear her call out for help.

17. What additional resources will you need? Why?

18. Describe how to set up a landing zone for the helicopter.

19. Once the tree is stabilized and no other hazards exist, what care can you provide to the patient while you wait for the EMTs to arrive?

APPENDIX 1

AMERICAN HEART ASSOCIATION
Skill Performance Sheets

Work in small groups to practice caring for patients who need artificial ventilation and CPR. Practice on CPR manikins until each member of your group achieves a "perfect score."

Skill Performance Sheet
Adult One-Rescuer CPR

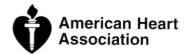

American Heart Association

Student Name _____ Date _____

Performance Guidelines	Performed
1. Establish unresponsiveness. Activate the EMS system.	
2. Open airway (head tilt–chin lift or jaw thrust). Check breathing (look, listen, feel).*	
3. Give 2 slow breaths (1 1/2 to 2 seconds per breath), watch chest rise, allow for exhalation between breaths.	
4. Check carotid pulse. If breathing is absent but pulse is present, provide rescue breathing (1 breath every 5 seconds, about 12 breaths per minute).	
5. If no pulse, give cycles of 15 chest compressions (rate, 80 to 100 compressions per minute) followed by 2 slow breaths.	
6. After 4 cycles of 15:2 (about 1 minute), check pulse.* If no pulse, continue 15:2 cycle beginning with chest compressions.	

*If victim is breathing or resumes effective breathing, place in recovery position.

Comments _____

_____

_____

Instructor _____

Circle one: Complete   Needs more practice

Reproduced with permission.
© *Basic Life Support Heartsaver Guide,* 1993
Copyright American Heart Association.

Skill Performance Sheet
Adult Two-Rescuer CPR

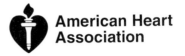

American Heart Association

Student Name _____ Date _____

Performance Guidelines	Performed
1. Establish unresponsiveness. EMS system has been activated.	
RESCUER 1	
2. Open airway (head tilt–chin lift or jaw thrust). Check breathing (look, listen, feel).*	
3. Give 2 slow breaths (1 ½ to 2 seconds per breath), watch chest rise, allow for exhalation between breaths.	
4. Check carotid pulse.	
RESCUER 2	
5. If no pulse, give cycles of 5 chest compressions (rate, 80 to 100 compressions per minute) followed by 1 slow breath by Rescuer 1.	
6. After 1 minute of rescue support, check pulse.* If no pulse, continue 5:1 cycles.	

*If victim is breathing or resumes effective breathing, place in recovery position.

Comments _____

_____

_____

Instructor _____

Circle one: Complete   Needs more practice

Reproduced with permission.
© *Basic Life Support Heartsaver Guide,* 1993
Copyright American Heart Association.

Skill Performance Sheet
Adult Foreign-Body Airway Obstruction— Conscious

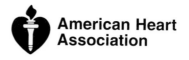

American Heart Association

Student Name _____ Date _____

Performance Guidelines	Performed
1. Ask "Are you choking?"	
2. Give abdominal thrusts (chest thrusts for pregnant or obese victim).	
3. Repeat thrusts until effective or victim becomes unconscious.	
Adult Foreign-Body Airway Obstruction— Victim Becomes Unconscious	
4. Activate the EMS system.	
5. Perform a tongue-jaw lift followed by a finger sweep to remove the object.	
6. Open airway and try to ventilate; if still obstructed, reposition head and try to ventilate again.	
7. Give up to 5 abdominal thrusts.	
8. Repeat steps 5 through 7 until effective.*	

*If victim is breathing or resumes effective breathing, place in recovery position.

Comments _____

_____

_____

Instructor _____

Circle one: Complete   Needs more practice

Reproduced with permission.
© *Basic Life Support Heartsaver Guide,* 1993
Copyright American Heart Association.

Skill Performance Sheet
Adult Foreign-Body Airway Obstruction— Unconscious

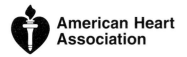

American Heart Association

Student Name _____ Date _____

Performance Guidelines	Performed
1. Establish unresponsiveness. Activate the EMS system.	
2. Open airway and try to ventilate; if still obstructed, reposition head and try to ventilate again.	
3. Give up to 5 abdominal thrusts.	
4. Perform a tongue-jaw lift followed by a finger sweep to remove the object.	
5. Repeat steps 2 through 4 until effective.*	

*If victim is breathing or resumes effective breathing, place in recovery position.

Comments _____

_____

_____

Instructor _____

Circle one: Complete   Needs more practice

Reproduced with permission.
© *Basic Life Support Heartsaver Guide,* 1993
Copyright American Heart Association.

Skill Performance Sheet
Child One-Rescuer CPR

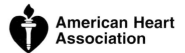 **American Heart Association**

Student Name _____ Date _____

Performance Guidelines	Performed
1. Establish unresponsiveness. If second rescuer is available, have him or her activate the EMS system.	
2. Open airway (head tilt–chin lift or jaw thrust). Check breathing (look, listen, feel).*	
3. Give 2 slow breaths (1 to 1 1/2 seconds per breath), watch chest rise, allow for exhalation between breaths.	
4. Check carotid pulse. If breathing is absent but pulse is present, provide rescue breathing (1 breath every 3 seconds, about 20 breaths per minute).	
5. If no pulse, give 5 chest compressions (100 compressions per minute), open airway, and provide 1 slow breath. Repeat this cycle.	
6. After about 1 minute of rescue support, check pulse.* If rescuer is alone, activate the EMS system. If no pulse, continue 5:1 cycles.	

*If victim is breathing or resumes effective breathing, place in recovery position.

Comments _____

_____

_____

Instructor _____

Circle one: Complete   Needs more practice

Reproduced with permission.
© *Basic Life Support Heartsaver Guide,* 1993
Copyright American Heart Association.

Skill Performance Sheet
Child Foreign-Body Airway Obstruction— Conscious

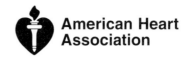 **American Heart Association**

Student Name _____ Date _____

Performance Guidelines	Performed
1. Ask "Are you choking?"	
2. Give abdominal thrusts.	
3. Repeat thrusts until effective or victim becomes unconscious.	
Child Foreign-Body Airway Obstruction— Victim Becomes Unconscious	
4. If second rescuer is available, have him or her activate the EMS system.	
5. Perform a tongue-jaw lift, and if you see the object, perform a finger sweep to remove it.	
6. Open airway and try to ventilate; if still obstructed, reposition head and try to ventilate again.	
7. Give up to 5 abdominal thrusts.	
8. Repeat steps 5 through 7 until effective.*	
9. If airway obstruction is not relieved after about 1 minute, activate the EMS system.	

*If victim is breathing or resumes effective breathing, place in recovery position.

Comments _____

_____

_____

Instructor _____

Circle one: Complete   Needs more practice

Reproduced with permission.
© *Basic Life Support Heartsaver Guide,* 1993
Copyright American Heart Association.

Skill Performance Sheet
Child Foreign-Body
Airway Obstruction—
Unconscious

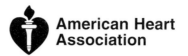

American Heart Association

Student Name _____ Date _____

Performance Guidelines	Performed
1. Establish unresponsiveness. If second rescuer is available, have him or her activate the EMS system.	
2. Open airway and try to ventilate; if still obstructed, reposition head and try to ventilate again.	
3. Give up to 5 abdominal thrusts.	
4. Perform a tongue-jaw lift, and if you see the object, perform a finger sweep to remove it.	
5. Repeat steps 2 through 4 until effective.*	
6. If airway obstruction is not relieved after about 1 minute, activate the EMS system.	

*If victim is breathing or resumes effective breathing, place in recovery position.

Comments _____

_____

_____

Instructor _____

Circle one: Complete   Needs more practice

Reproduced with permission.
© *Basic Life Support Heartsaver Guide,* 1993
Copyright American Heart Association.

Skill Performance Sheet
Infant One-Rescuer CPR

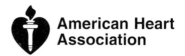 American Heart Association

Student Name _____ Date _____

Performance Guidelines	Performed
1. Establish unresponsiveness. If second rescuer is available, have him or her activate the EMS system.	
2. Open airway (head tilt–chin lift or jaw thrust). Check breathing (look, listen, feel).*	
3. Give 2 slow breaths (1 to 1 1/2 seconds per breath), watch chest rise, allow for exhalation between breaths.	
4. Check brachial pulse. If breathing is absent but pulse is present, provide rescue breathing (1 breath every 3 seconds, about 20 breaths per minute).	
5. If no pulse, give cycles of 5 chest compressions (rate, at least 100 compressions per minute) followed by 1 slow breath.	
6. After about 1 minute of rescue support, check pulse.* If rescuer is alone, activate the EMS system. If no pulse, continue 5:1 cycles.	

*If victim is breathing or resumes effective breathing, place in recovery position.

Comments _____

_____

_____

Instructor _____

Circle one: Complete   Needs more practice

Reproduced with permission.
© *Basic Life Support Heartsaver Guide,* 1993
Copyright American Heart Association.

Skill Performance Sheet
Infant Foreign-Body
Airway Obstruction—
Conscious

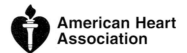

American Heart Association

Student Name _____   Date _____

Performance Guidelines	Performed
1. Confirm complete airway obstruction. Check for serious breathing difficulty, ineffective cough, *no* strong cry.	
2. Give up to 5 back blows and 5 chest thrusts.	
3. Repeat step 2 until effective or victim becomes unconscious.	
Infant Foreign-Body Airway Obstruction— Victim Becomes Unconscious	
4. If second rescuer is available, have him or her activate the EMS system.	
5. Perform a tongue-jaw lift, and if you see the object, perform a finger sweep to remove it.	
6. Open airway and try to ventilate; if still obstructed, reposition head and try to ventilate again.	
7. Give up to 5 back blows and 5 chest thrusts.	
8. Repeat steps 5 through 7 until effective.*	
9. If airway obstruction is not relieved after about 1 minute, activate the EMS system.	

*If victim is breathing or resumes effective breathing, place in recovery position.

Comments _____

_____

_____

Instructor _____

Circle one: Complete   Needs more practice

Reproduced with permission.
© *Basic Life Support Heartsaver Guide,* 1993
Copyright American Heart Association.

Skill Performance Sheet
Infant Foreign-Body
Airway Obstruction—
Unconscious

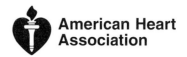

American Heart Association

Student Name _____ Date _____

Performance Guidelines	Performed
1. Establish unresponsiveness. If second rescuer is available, have him or her activate the EMS system.	
2. Open airway and try to ventilate; if still obstructed, reposition head and try to ventilate again.	
3. Give up to 5 back blows and 5 chest thrusts.	
4. Perform a tongue-jaw lift, and if you see the object, perform a finger sweep to remove it.	
5. Repeat steps 2 through 4 until effective.*	
6. If airway obstruction is not relieved after about 1 minute, activate the EMS system.	

*If victim is breathing or resumes effective breathing, place in recovery position.

Comments _____

_____

_____

Instructor _____

Circle one: Complete   Needs more practice

Reproduced with permission.
© *Basic Life Support Heartsaver Guide,* 1993
Copyright American Heart Association.

APPENDIX 2

FIRST RESPONDER: A SKILLS APPROACH
Skill Summary Sheets

Work in small groups to practice caring for patients until each member of your group achieves a "perfect score." Note that the daggers (†) below indicate skills supplemental to the DOT 1995 "First Responder: National Standard Curriculum" and may not be required of First Responders in your EMS system. Be sure you learn and follow all state and local protocols.

FIRST RESPONDER: A SKILLS APPROACH
SKILL SUMMARY SHEETS

MANUAL STABILIZATION
OF A TRAUMA PATIENT'S HEAD AND NECK

▼	SKILL SUMMARY	Check If Performed
1	Take BSI precautions.	
2	Tell the patient to stay very still.	
3	Place your hands on both sides of the patient's head and hold it firmly and steadily in a neutral, in-line position.	
4	Maintain manual stabilization until the patient is completely immobilized.	
NOTE: If your patient's head is not already in a neutral, in-line position when you begin, gently guide it there. If there is any pain or if you feel resistance, stop immediately and stabilize the head in the position in which it was found.		

SUCTIONING

▼	SKILL SUMMARY	Check If Performed
1	Take BSI precautions.	
2	Prepare the suction device.	
3	Select the correct type of catheter for your patient.	
4	Without suction, insert the catheter to the base of the patient's tongue.	
5	Apply suction while moving the catheter from side to side.	
6	Suction for up to 15 seconds in an adult (10 seconds in a child and 5 seconds in an infant).	
NOTE: If decreased heart rate is observed in an infant you are suctioning, stop and reapply oxygen or ventilate for at least 30 seconds prior to suctioning again.		

Student's Name _____ Date _____

THE OROPHARYNGEAL AIRWAY

	SKILL SUMMARY	Check If Performed
1	Take BSI precautions.	
2	Select the proper size airway.	
3	Open the patient's mouth. If necessary, use the cross-finger technique.	
4	In an adult, insert the airway upside down, with the top pointing toward the roof of the patient's mouth.	
5	Advance the airway gently until you meet resistance.	
6	Rotate the airway 180° clockwise while you continue to advance it, until the flange rests on the patient's front teeth.	
NOTE: In an infant or child, use a tongue depressor and insert the airway in its normal upright position. Do not rotate it.		

THE NASOPHARYNGEAL AIRWAY

	SKILL SUMMARY	Check If Performed
1	Take BSI precautions.	
2	Select the proper size airway.	
3	Lubricate the device with a sterile, water-soluble lubricant.	
4	Insert the airway posteriorly, with the beveled end toward the septum when it is inserted in the right nostril.	
5	Advance the airway gently and close to the midline along the floor of the nostril and straight back into the nasopharynx.	
NOTE: If the airway cannot be inserted in one nostril, try the other nostril.		

Student's Name _____ Date _____

FIRST RESPONDER: A SKILLS APPROACH
SKILL SUMMARY SHEETS

OXYGEN ADMINISTRATION

▼ SKILL SUMMARY	Check If Performed
1 Take BSI precautions.	
2 Identify the cylinder as oxygen, and remove the protective seal from the tank.	
3 Crack the main cylinder for one second to remove dust and debris.	
4 Place the yoke of the regulator over the cylinder valve and align the pins.	
5 Hand-tighten the T-screw on the regulator.	
6 Open the main cylinder valve to check the pressure.	
7 Attach the proper delivery device (nonrebreather mask or nasal cannula) to the regulator.	
8 Adjust the flow meter to the appropriate liter flow (nonrebreather mask—15 liters per minute; nasal cannula—no more than 6 liters per minute).	
9 Apply the oxygen delivery device to the patient.	
NOTE: When you are ready to discontinue oxygen administration, remove the device from the patient. Then shut off the control valve until liter flow is at zero. Shut off the main cylinder valve. Then bleed the valves by leaving the control valve open until the needle or ball indicator returns to zero.	

APPENDIX 2 • SKILL SUMMARY SHEETS **279**

FIRST RESPONDER: A SKILLS APPROACH
SKILL SUMMARY SHEETS

EXTERNAL BLEEDING CONTROL

	SKILL SUMMARY	Check If Performed
1	Take BSI precautions.	
2	Apply direct pressure to the bleeding wound.	
3	Elevate the extremity, but only if there is no major injury to the underlying muscle or bone.	
4	Reassess bleeding. If bleeding has not stopped, then apply additional pressure as needed.	
5	If bleeding continues, apply pressure to the arterial pulse point above the wound on the injured extremity.	
6	Reassess bleeding. When bleeding is under control, bandage the wound appropriately.	

SHOCK MANAGEMENT

	SKILL SUMMARY	Check If Performed
1	Take BSI precautions.	
2	Maintain an open airway in the patient. If breathing is adequate, administer oxygen by way of a nonrebreather mask. Be prepared to provide artificial ventilation, if needed.	
3	Prevent any further blood loss.	
4	Position the patient properly.	
5	Keep the patient warm, but do not overheat him or her.	
6	Provide care for specific injuries while waiting for EMS crews to arrive.	
NOTE: Comfort, calm, and reassure the patient while you wait for transport. Be sure to withhold all food and drink.		

Student's Name _____ Date _____

FIRST RESPONDER: A SKILLS APPROACH
SKILL SUMMARY SHEETS

SPLINTING

	SKILL SUMMARY	Check If Performed
1	Take BSI precautions.	
2	Instruct another First Responder or a helper to apply manual stabilization to the injured extremity.	
3	Assess pulse, movement, and sensation below the injury site.	
4	Cut away clothing to expose the injury to the extremity.	
5	After controlling bleeding, place a sterile dressing over open wounds, if any.	
6	If there is severe deformity, absence of a pulse, or cyanosis in the extremity, align it with gentle manual traction. Maintain it until the limb is completely immobilized.	
7	Measure the splint, and pad it appropriately.	
8	For a long-bone injury, apply the splint so that the joints above and below the injury site are immobilized. For a joint injury, apply the splint so the bones above and below the injury site are immobilized.	
9	Secure the injured extremity to the splint.	
10	Reassess pulse, movement, and sensation in the extremity every 15 minutes and record your findings.	
NOTE: If the limb is severely deformed by the injury, or if the limb has no pulse or is cyanotic below the injury site, then align it with gentle manual traction. If there is pain or grating, stop pulling immediately.		

APPENDIX 3

Practice Scenarios

Bring together all the knowledge and skills you have acquired in this course. Work with partners or in small groups to decide what you would do for each scenario below.

1. Your patient is in bed, unresponsive. There is shortness of breath, unusually slow pulse, and bluish, cool, damp skin. After you are told the patient is terminally ill, you are given a DNA order by his son.

2. The alarmed parents say the infant is "too quiet." The babysitter noticed nothing unusual, they report. The baby appears to you to be sleepy and pale.

3. Your partner has been exceptionally irritable lately. He seems to be either snapping at someone—including patients—or daydreaming. He has been late to the job several times and refuses to break with the rest of the crew.

4. Your adult patient has a painful, swollen, deformed injury to the lower right arm with pulselessness below the injury site.

5. A 40-year-old woman is unconscious. She has old and new bruises on her face, arms, chest, stomach, and legs. Her husband, who is nearby, appears to be unable to stand still or meet your partner's eyes.

6. The eight-year-old boy has been lost on the mountain in the woods for nine hours. Sunset was five hours ago. When you find him, he is wearing only a tee shirt and shorts.

7. Your 35-year-old patient, who has been sunning all day on the beach. When you reach her, you find that her skin is dry and hot and she is unresponsive.

8. A 10-year-old girl steps on a rusty five-inch nail, which goes completely through her foot.

9. Your patient was ejected through the windshield of a moving vehicle. She is now unresponsive and showing signs of breathing difficulty.

10. Your patient is an 18-year-old woman who 15 minutes before opened her front door, stepped onto a sheet of ice, and fell down five concrete steps. She said she landed on her "tail bone," which was and is still very painful.

11. The patient is a five-year-old boy with severe breathing difficulty. You suspect a partial foreign body airway obstruction.

12. Your 18-year-old patient has a stab wound to the neck. He is bleeding profusely.

13. Your patient has sliced off the index finger of her left hand and partially severed the thumb with a jigsaw. She is bleeding profusely.

14. It is summer and you and your partner are patrolling the lake's public beach when you see an adult male swimmer who appears to be having difficulty in the water about 50 feet from shore.

15. Your patient has been shot in the chest in a gang incident. The bullet wound entered through his back just below the scapula.

16. The patient fell, feet first, approximately 18 feet onto concrete. He is pale and unresponsive with obvious deformity to his right thigh.

17. Your 30-year-old patient was in a car crash. Both forearms are painful, swollen, and deformed. She also has suffered a blow to her forehead. On the AVPU scale, your patient is verbal. Radial pulse is weak. Skin condition is pale, cool, moist.

18. Your patient is a 19-year-old male who was thrown from a pickup truck that rolled over several times. The driver is dead. Your patient says he is fine and wants to go home now.

19. You are restocking your supplies when you are called to respond to a "fist fight" in front of the bar on the corner of Main and Connor. You must decide quickly on the personal protective equipment to take with you.

20. An 88-year-old woman tripped over her telephone cord and fell on the floor. She is complaining of severe pain in her left hip and thigh.

21. Suddenly the firefighters present you with a 70-year-old woman who has partial-thickness burns on her arms and chest. The patient has soot around her nostrils and mouth.

22. Your patient's face and neck have been slashed with a razor. There is profuse bleeding from the neck.

23. You are called to a "delivery in progress." When you arrive on scene, you are told that the baby is not due for another six weeks.

24. You are watching a game of stick ball when you see a speeding car sideswipe one of the players and race away. The boy—10 years old—was spun into the air, hit the hood of a parked car, and slid to the ground.

25. A diner performs abdominal thrusts on a man who is choking. After several thrusts, you see the patient lose consciousness and drop to the floor. No one is doing anything to help him.

26. The weather is overcast and cold at the triathlon. The contestants finished the swim portion of the race, and they are getting on their bikes to start the second event. One contestant, however, is sitting on the ground, shivering and pale.

27. A farm worker has been found unresponsive in the immediate area of a manure pit.

28. You are shopping at Macy's when you see a man clutch at his left arm and fall to the ground unconscious.

29. A 20-year-old female has just given birth. The infant is blue and limp, and the mother appears to have lost an excessive amount of blood.

30. You are exiting the "Y" where you are a swim instructor when a very young woman in obvious distress is carried through the door by an older male. He looks at you and says, "Help, the baby is coming!"

31. The woman is 22 with contractions that are four minutes apart and 45 seconds each. This is her first baby. She is 30 minutes from the nearest medical facility.

32. You are dispatched to the skateboard park for a 13-year-old male who fell off one of the ramps directly onto his head. He is complaining of neck pain.

33. You are caring for a 13-year-old girl who caught her fingers in a car door as it was slammed shut. The girl is screaming in pain. Her parents, who are trying to comfort her, are very upset. Her hand appears to be swelling and bleeding, and the fingertips are blue. There is a large puncture wound on the upper palm.

34. You have just helped a new mother deliver her baby. The newborn's pulse rate is less than 100 beats per minute.

35. Your patient is short of breath. His breathing is rapid, and he is experiencing tingling around his mouth and fingertips.

36. You are called to the scene of a drowning. When you arrive, you see an adult male performing CPR incorrectly on a supine, six-year-old child.

37. You are called to an industrial plant with a report of a gas leak and five workers down. You will arrive on the scene about five minutes before the fire service and hazmat teams.

38. You are called to an "auto versus pole." The 82-year-old driver is alert but has pain in her chest from striking the steering wheel. She has no memory of how the crash occurred.

39. You are called to a baby who appears to be dead in her crib. Her parents are demanding that you do something to help her.

40. You are called to a "man having an asthma attack." He tells you that he just has to "get a shot" at the hospital "like last time."

41. You are approaching the scene of a vehicle collision involving a tanker truck and a small pickup. Dispatch reports that the crash may involve a hazardous materials spill.

42. You have been called to a "man down" in an alley behind a high-rise office building. He smells of alcohol and cannot be roused when you call out to him.

43. Your patient is a 66-year-old male who is having chest pain. He is pale and sweaty. He has already taken several nitroglycerin tablets.

44. Your patient is 8 years old. Her mother says she is having an acute asthma attack. The child has irregular breathing, high-pitched breathing sounds, and a rapid pulse.

45. A 46-year-old male has abdominal pain. He suddenly vomits a large amount of bright, red blood and becomes pale and sweaty.

46. You are alone on the scene of a vehicle collision involving 20 or more people. Rescue vehicles will have a difficult time getting through the traffic.

47. It is a hot, sunny day. You are patrolling the shopping mall parking lot when you see a baby locked alone in a car. The baby—about one year old—is wearing a buttoned up sweater over a long-sleeve shirt, long pants, socks, and shoes. The baby appears to have hot, moist skin.

48. Your patient is a 40-year-old woman who has just been beaten and robbed. You suspect she also may have been raped.

49. Your 21-month-old patient has ingested an unknown quantity of aspirin tablets. The child has a white powder around his mouth. He is alert, happy, and interacting normally with his mother and his environment.

50. Your patient was chopping wood into tinder when "something" flew into his left eye. He has been running tap water over his eye. He can no longer open it.

51. An adult male is reported to have had sharp abdominal pain for several hours. He has taken several doses of an over-the-counter antacid but has had no relief. He is in mild distress. His skin is cool and moist.

52. An adult female, possibly in her 30s, has been found lying in bed, cyanotic, and unresponsive, with a slow respiratory rate. There is drug paraphernalia nearby.

53. An 86-year-old man awoke with shortness of breath one hour ago. He is sitting straight up and appears to be in severe distress. He looks fatigued and is unable to speak.

54. You have just arrived with the fire department on the scene of a fire in an office building. It appears that over 50 people have been injured by smoke inhalation, burns, or falls while trying to escape.

55. After starting a new prescription for a urinary tract infection, a woman complains of nausea, vomiting, abdominal cramps, and diarrhea.

56. A teenager was checking the engine radiator when a jet of boiling hot steam and water hits her face. Her mother is frantic as she pulls you to the back of the house where you hear screams of pain.

57. A man in a wheelchair is whooping loudly as he careens up and down the street, bashing into parked cars, and generally terrorizing the neighborhood. As you watch, the man speeds toward a passerby, misses hitting her only by inches, and U-turns back towards you.

58. A day-care-center supervisor reports that six children are vomiting and appear to have abdominal pain and cramping. The teaching assistant also does not feel well.

59. You have responded to a motor-vehicle collision. Your unresponsive patient's mid-size car has been hit from the rear in traffic that was moving at about 30 mph. He is still wearing his lap belt. There appears to be no headrest.

60. A 70-year-old woman was found by her sons in bed, unable to speak and unable to move the right side of her body. She has a slow pulse and rapid respirations.

61. A 63-year-old is mowing the lawn when very suddenly she finds that she "can't breathe."

62. A 35-year-old male is "vomiting blood." The patient is very pale and says he is dizzy and might "pass out."

63. A 31-year-old male fell off his bicycle during a road race. The patient is standing, cradling his right arm close to his body. It appears that there is some deformity of the right clavicle.

64. A 30-year-old woman has fallen from the roof of her two-story home onto newly turned earth. She is flat on her back and unresponsive.

65. A 30-year-old male accidentally shot himself with his own hand gun. He has a small entry wound in the upper right thigh. He is awake and alert but appears to be getting pale.

66. A 27-year-old male, reported to have a seizure, seems unable or unwilling to speak. He is slightly combative and uncooperative.

67. A 22-year-old athlete complains of chest pain about 20 minutes after a basketball game. She feels short of breath and markedly anxious.

68. A 17-year-old female has "slashed her wrists" in the locker room of the high school gym. She is upset, crying, and uncooperative. She will not answer any of your questions.

69. A 13-year-old and his father are eating hot dogs "with the works" when the youngster has a sudden onset of shortness of breath and facial itching, flushing, and swelling. He also has a cough, hoarseness, and noisy breathing.

70. A 70-year-old woman tells you she was taking a shower, when she realized her left arm and hand were—and still are—completely numb. She appears to be lethargic and slightly confused. She is wearing a Medic Alert bracelet that indicates she has diabetes.